Clinical Biochemistry

Contemporary Theories and Techniques

VOLUME 1

Edited by
HERBERT E. SPIEGEL

Department of Clinical Laboratory Research
Hoffmann-La Roche Inc.
Nutley, New Jersey

1981

ACADEMIC PRESS

A Subsidiary of Harcourt Brace Jovanovich, Publishers

New York   London
Paris   San Diego   San Francisco   São Paulo
Sydney   Tokyo   Toronto

ACADEMIC PRESS, INC.
111 Fifth Avenue, New York, New York 10003

United Kingdom Edition published by
ACADEMIC PRESS, INC. (LONDON) LTD.
24/28 Oval Road, London NW1   7DX

Library of Congress Cataloging in Publication Data
Main entry under title:

Clinical biochemistry.

    Includes bibliographies and index.
    1. Chemistry, Clinical. 2. Biological
chemistry.   I. Spiegel, Herbert E. [DNLM:
1. Chemistry, Clinical. QY 90 C6406]
RB40.C56   616.07'56   81-14933
ISBN 0-12-657101-5 (v. 1)   AACR2

PRINTED IN THE UNITED STATES OF AMERICA

81 82 83 84   9 8 7 6 5 4 3 2 1

Contents

1 Laboratory Management for Clinical Chemists

THOMAS C. ROBINSON and MAX E. CHILCOTE

2 Laboratory Safety and Environmental Monitoring

WESLEY R. VAN PELT

3   Criteria for Kit Selection in Clinical Chemistry

JAMES E. LOGAN

4   Mathematics in Clinical Chemistry

WENDELL T. CARAWAY

5   Blood Gases, pH, and Acid–Base Balance

NORMAN LASKER

6 Autoimmune Disease

GLORIA A. MARCANTUONO

7 Specific Proteins in Plasma, Cerebrospinal Fluid, Urine, and Other Biological Fluids

LAWRENCE M. KILLINGSWORTH and CAROL E. KILLINGSWORTH

List of Contributors

Numbers in parentheses indicate the pages on which the authors' contributions begin.

Wendell T. Caraway (87), Laboratories of McLaren General Hospital, and St. Joseph Hospital, Flint, Michigan 48502.

Max E. Chilcote (1), Erie County Laboratory, Erie County Medical Center, Buffalo, New York 14215

Carol E. Killingsworth (187), Clinical Chemistry and Immunology Laboratories, Department of Pathology, Sacred Heart Medical Center, Spokane, Washington 99220

Lawrence M. Killingsworth (187), Clinical Chemistry and Immunology Laboratories, Department of Pathology, Sacred Heart Medical Center, Spokane, Washington 99220

Norman Lasker (123), Department of Medicine, Division of Nephrology, CMDNJ–New Jersey Medical School, Newark, New Jersey 07103

James E. Logan (43), Laboratory Center for Disease Control, Bureau of Medical Biochemistry, Health Protection Branch, Ottawa, Ontario, Canada K1A 0L2

Gloria A. Marcantuono (157), Department of Microbiology and Immunology, The Mountainside Hospital, Montclair, New Jersey 07042

*Thomas C. Robinson** (1), Erie County Laboratory, Erie County Medical Center, Buffalo, New York 14215

Wesley R. Van Pelt (23), Industrial Hygiene Group, Department of Corporate, Environmental, and Safety Affairs, Hoffmann-La Roche, Inc., Nutley, New Jersey 07110

---

* Present address: Albert B. Chandler Medical Center, College of Allied Health Professions, University of Kentucky, Lexington, Kentucky 40536

Preface

The purpose of this treatise is to give formal expression to the ideas and philosophies of scientific leaders in the many disciplines related to clinical chemistry. Every attempt has been made by the editor to preserve the individual style of the contributor. It is hoped that these individualized presentations will provide the reader with the impression of conducting a dialogue with the contributor.

A further intent of this volume is to supplement the existing textbooks of clinical chemistry and biochemistry by providing areas of emphasis, such as the biochemistry of aging, managerial techniques, the evaluation of kits, and autoimmune disease, which are usually not emphasized in standard clinical chemistry texts. Where possible, details are de-emphasized in favor of overall concepts and philosophy. Speculation and interpretation by the contributors have been encouraged with the idea that these will be stimulating to the reader.

We trust we have designed a collection of essays to acquaint the reader with the wide spectrum of sciences that is called clinical chemistry.

Herbert E. Spiegel

Acknowledgments

I wish to acknowledge the cooperation and talents of the many contributors to this volume. In addition, it would be most appropriate to acknowledge the tireless efforts of my secretary, Joan Marks. Finally, I would like to express my appreciation to my wife, Joanne, and to my family for the encouragement without which this volume would not have been possible.

Laboratory Management for Clinical Chemists

THOMAS C. ROBINSON
AND MAX E. CHILCOTE

I. INTRODUCTION

The reader must, in our opinion, be told immediately of our interpretation (view) of the intent (guiding philosophy) and the practical limitations of a single chapter on laboratory management. The available literature is greater in both volume and value to the clinical chemist than is immediately apparent from the background education and training of most clinical chemists. In brief, laboratory management is people management just as for most businesses. People budgets, for example, constitute by far the largest share of total budgets. Thus, the clinical chemist must learn to work with individuals both above and below in the organizational structure of the clinical laboratory in order to provide the optimum laboratory

CLINICAL BIOCHEMISTRY
Contemporary Theories and Techniques, Vol. 1

services at the lowest cost possible. Cost effectiveness is a term you will have to live with and attempt to redefine to your administrative colleagues. The many topics covered by this subject demand entire books—notice the term books instead of book. Please refer to references (Bennington, 1977; Lundberg, 1975) for the more comprehensive discussions necessary to your ability to provide as close to the optimum laboratory services we all desire. Other texts on the subject will probably continue to appear as the necessity for better cost-effective management becomes more widely appreciated.

As the reader may well, and should indeed, wonder why the following emphasis on administrative theory, this introduction addresses that problem. Government has brought to the fore the professionally trained administrator with business practice and/or legal training with perhaps little if any training in the natural or physical sciences. Their training leads many, if not most, of them to believe that tight, logical, disciplined thinking can solve any problem with the aid of only a minimal exposure to the background of the problem. They can be expected to ask questions such as: "Why do you insist on using highly paid Medical Technologists to perform the routine procedures? If given detailed instructions, can't just one Medical Technician supervise a room full of high school graduates?" Or, "Why must your quality control program use so many costly control sera (or such expensive vacutainers)? After all, Company A products are so much cheaper, and I know Hospital Z uses them. Why do you insist on Company B?" In brief, the elements of cost control are highly ingrained into their background, and are essential to sound business practice. In contrast, the correlation of very high quality clinical laboratory data, comparable and high quality interpretation, to high quality medical practice is entirely foreign to them. The gulf is background thinking (knowledge of the complexities involved in a modern clinical laboratory setting, decisions in setting priorities) between you, the clinical chemist, and them is very much deeper and broader than you may think. In brief, they are on the side of quantity and cost which you must battle to get near the quality you will desire. Thus, you must develop some understanding of their *raison d'etre*.

II. ORGANIZATIONAL ENVIRONMENT

The clinical laboratory is most often found in an institutional setting. Any institution contains an organizational structure and staff with people who interpret its goals and mission. It contains informal and formal lines of communications. Values and traditions are inescapable in the roles that each individual in the institution plays. Change is inherent in institutions. Leadership roles shift and technologies continue to improve.

The period in which we live in health care is confusing and complicated. Those in authority must provide order to the organization that we call the clinical laboratory, so that it can more effectively be managed. Management theory and skills generally are not a part of the educational preparation of most laboratory managers.

A. Organizational Theory

Organizational theory as we know it is a collection of theories. The literature of organizational theory contains many different approaches to describing organization and its management. This discussion is an overview of the most representative themes in the literature with the understanding that it is not all inclusive.

1. Classical School

Organization theory has its beginnings in *Scientific Management* (Taylor, 1911). This school, the Classical School, sees workers as motivated by economic reward only, and the collateral organization is defined through a *division of labor; highly specialized personnel;* and a *hierarchical authority structure*. Etzioni (1964) gives us the most succinct definition:

> Scientific Management combines a study of physical capabilities of a worker, as is still done (primarily by engineers) in time and motion studies, with an economic approach which views man as driven by the fear of hunger and the search for profit. The central tenet of the approach is that if material rewards are closely related to work efforts, the worker will respond with the maximum performance he is physically capable of (Etzioni, 1964).

Taylor's world deals with the worker and the machine as mutually related, and with proper rewards both achieve maximal response. This school sees the human body with a capability, as an example, for shoveling coal, and given the right environment and motivation, the optimum amount of coal can be shoveled.

A contemporary of Taylor, who reflects the same philosophic approach, was Max Weber (1947), a German sociologist who suggests bureaucracy as the "ideal type" of organization. Similar themes to Taylor surface in Weber—technical competence, the division of labor and specialization, hierarchy of authority, rules and standard operating procedures, and exact work duties and authority.

Both men describe what they saw; the capatalist systems of Germany and the United States. In the United States, in particular, it was a time when the government took a *laissez-faire* attitude. Decision-making was more decentralized than today, and collective bargaining was rare indeed. It was the time when the "captains of industry" had successfully contained their industrial empires with "managers."

Classical proponents remain. In more recent works, neoclassics have modified some of the original statements of the scientific school.

There are certain values that are crucial to management according to the neoclassics (Simon *et al.,* 1959).

1. *Accountability* is the responsibility of the supervisor to see that his directives are carried out and the responsibility of the supervised to carry them out. This augments the concept of control and the hierarchy authority system.
2. *Expertness and economy,* another concept, represents a more developed idea of the division of labor, and makes the case for removal of anciliary activities from all departments and establishment of service departments for greater effectiveness of purpose; e.g., centralized purchasing, typing, storeroom, etc.
3. The concept of *levels of conflict settlement* expands the hierarchical organization as a control group, and defines it also as a mechanism to resolve internal conflict. The most effective settlement of conflict is at the lowest levels within the structure.
4. *Program emphasis* is a way to prevent slow growth away from the original objectives of the organization. More privileges and perogatives are delegated to those departments of functions which are more central to the original objectives of the organization.
5. The *classical school* views the world through the rational use of formal organizational tools as the most effective way to achieve success in meeting the goals of the organization.

The bureaucratic orientation and the scientific approach was adequate until the 1930s. The traditional approach did not concern itself with the human elements and its effect on the organization to the success of goals mastery.

2. Human Relations School

The Human Relations School, a collection of several theorists, contributes the next major emphasis on the continuum of theory development.

The historical context of the time was radically different than the buoyancy of the turn-of-the-century. By the 1930s, government involvement and control, collective bargaining, and economic disaster dramatically altered everyone's view of the world and consequently, their view of organizations in that world.

As social science grew in its ability to measure, researchers conducted studies that shed light on the effectiveness of the more traditional approaches to management and, subsequently, questioned the assumptions of the classical school. The human or social relationship of a worker with his organizational environment was discovered.

The landmark study is one of a series under Elton Mayo known as the Hawthorne Studies. It had been considered, by the tenets of Scientific Management, that if the work environment was improved, then productivity would increase. In this experiment, better illumination was provided, and it was expected that individual worker productivity would improve. *The results contradict this assumption.* In fact, the improved environment and productivity are unrelated. With follow-up study, the researchers conclude that it is the group process that affects productivity (Roethlesberger and Dickson, 1939). Membership in the work group and the norms of the group are the key factors in productivity, not the physical environment.

In fact, in many groups, "an artificial restriction of output" is based on the belief by the groups that if they produce "naturally," then pay will be reduced or, worse, their jobs will disappear.

The Hawthorne studies and the Western Electric study sets the stage for the human relations school (Roethlesberger and Dickson conducted productivity studies at the Western Electric Plant in Chicago from 1927 to 1932.), which postulate that the level of production is established by social norms, and that physiological capacity is no longer accepted. Affection and respect of the work group determine worker productivity. *Economic rewards alone do not* significantly affect the output of the work. Workers do not react as individuals, but rather as group members.

The human relations approach mandates that managers necessarily alter their approach to management within organizations to include group dynamics; the way groups function. Understanding of the informal organization is a trait of a human relations manager and he *shifts toward* an employee orientation, communication, and *participative decision-making.*

Human relations managers attempt to obtain the most efficient organization by cultivating the human resource. The worker who meets his personal (can be group determined) need, is the happiest and, thus, most productive.

Douglas McGregor (1960), a leading proponent at this approach to management, using Maslow's hierarchy of needs as a theoretical base, postulate that the *self-actualized person* is *the most effective.* McGregor provides the best summary of the assumptions underlying two schools of thought, scientific management, theory X, and the human relations school, theory Y.

a. Assumptions of Theory X
1. The average human being has an inherent dislike of work and will avoid it.
2. Because of this human characteristic of dislike of work, most people must be directed and threatened with punishment to get them to achieve objectives of the organization.
3. The average human being prefers to be led, wants to avoid responsibility, has little drive, seeks security above all.

b. Assumptions of Theory Y
1. Work is as natural as play or rest.
2. External control and the threat of punishment are not the only means to motivate. Man will exercise self-direction toward objectives to which he is committed.
3. Commitment to objectives is a function of the rewards associated with their achievement.
4. Man seeks to accept responsibility.
5. The capacity to exercise a relatively high degree of imagination, ingenuity, and creativity in the solution of organizational problems is widely distributed in the population.
6. Under the conditions of modern industrial life, the intellectual potentialities of the average human being are only partially utilized.

The classical school emphasizes the organization, the structure itself toward success; whereas, the human approach stresses the happy organization as the most satisfying, thus effective.

The two share a common framework; i.e., goal directed. The organization's press for rationality and the search for human happiness are not mutually exclusive.

3. Recent Theoretical Constructs

There are several more recent attempts to provide an expanded view of organization. These are labeled as the structuralist approach, and include several subgroups, including the contingency approach and the systems approach to organizations. Woodward (1965) and Katz and Kahn (1966) are excellent references in which to view the fields and attempt to interface the organization and its task environment.

The philosophical base of these approaches is that the nature of the organization's technology, its tasks, its staff, and its structure inter-relate and that change in one area impacts directly on another—much like an organizational ecological balance.

B. Functions and Principles of Management

Several concepts of management were documented by the original theorists. Many are considered current and one can readily recognize them in modern organizations and in particular in laboratory medicine.

What are the responsibilities of management? The acronym POSD-CORB aids in the enumeration of these functions.

1. *Planning.* Whether the mission is predetermined or determined by the manager, planning is the process of determining what needs to be done in the short run and, importantly, in the long run, i.e., plan objectives to meet the mission.
2. *Organizing.* The manager establishes a formal structure of authority of work-groups subject to that authority to meet the objectives.
3. *Staffing.* The manager hires and trains personnel to do the tasks of the organization.
4. *Directing.* The manager makes decisions continuously and tells the staff what tasks must be done to meet the objectives.
5. *Coordinating.* The manager guides these functions in an orderly sequence so as to meet the objectives.
6. *Reporting.* The manager must be informed of the measures of productivity, so as to evaluate for himself and the success the organization has in meeting its objectives.
7. *Budgeting.* The manager provides fiscal resources in order to obtain the resources, human and physical, to meet the objectives.

In order to successfully complete those functions, scientific managers employ several principles—the principles of management.

1. *Principles of unity of command.* Each subordinate is accountable to one and only one superior. More than one boss creates confusion resulting in inaction or inappropriate action.
2. *Principle of span of control.* One supervisor is responsible for 5–6 subordinates. Too many employees makes for loss of control, and thus ineffective leadership.
3. *Principle of delegation.* Delegation is the process by which a manager assigns responsibility, grants authority, and creates accountability. A good manager cannot do every task, and must assign some to others.
4. *The principle of the scalar chain.* There is an uninterrupted flow of authority through the organization. The chain of command links each supervisor at each level with his supervisor, allowing communication of information and delegation of authority.
5. *Role of staff and line.* Managers use staff to advise and line supervisors to command.

These are by no means complete nor is there a master list by which one can live.

The process of management by necessity begins with a delineation of objectives, and systematically with an evaluation that tells how well they were accomplished. The manager in the planning and decision-making process considers the central issue—one's original objectives.

"Management by objectives" (MBO), a phrase in recent use by managers, simply means that every person in the organization has a specific, realistic, and measurable objective consistent with the mission of the organization (Odiorne, 1965).

Health care institutions, like clinical laboratories, have the overriding mission of better patient care. The manager, in his decisions, insures that the activities of the departments and sections are compatable with that mission.

MBO has its roots in the human relations school. MBO is applied through the establishment of common goals, and a time frame to meet them is established by the manager in conjunction with his superior. The manager delineates a set of objectives individually with each subordinate which determines role behavior. All participants undertake the achievement of the planned goals. Near the end of the time frame, the actual performance of the individuals involved is measured against their individual goals. Achievements are discussed between subordinate and superior, and adjustment is made to either the objectives, goals, or the resources. This cycle is repeated.

Whether one does or can operate through MBO in the clinical laboratory, this theoretical construct does underscore the importance of clarification of objectives and subsequent action and decision-making (management) by these objectives rather than management by crisis.

III. MANAGEMENT SYSTEMS OF A CLINICAL CHEMISTRY LABORATORY

A. Clinical Laboratory as a System

Fanshel and Bush (1970) are two of many who describe health care as a system:

> To conceive of health services as a system is an analytical tool useful for rational planning. Thus, we say that the health system has a structure in which people and other resources are grouped together into sub-systems (programs, institutions, etc.) for the purpose of delivering all types of health services (environmental, financial, etc.). The health system also has a functional relation to the environment about it

(such as nonhealth governmental agencies and organized consumers). The performance of the system relates the output to the input to the activities performed by the
various structural elements (Fanshel and Bush, 1970).

If we focus our thesis sharper, a hospital as a singular organization
composes a system. The clinical laboratory and its components, including
a clinical chemistry laboratory, each represent a system.

The administrator or manager within that system needs, therefore, to
recognize the balance of components within that system.

The components that shape the organizational subsystem called the
clinical chemistry laboratory are interrelated inextricably to one another.
As a laboratory manager, one must, therefore, understand the relationship of the tasks, the technology, the people, and the structure of his
system.

What change occurs will affect each area. For example, the installation
of a laboratory computer represents a change in the manner the laboratory achieves its goals, i.e., generation of data to the clinician (for better
health care). This means substantial structural and human consequences.
Work units are regrouped, certain clerical and technical personnel are no
longer needed; new purchasing arrangements must be made; and new
technology must be mastered to operate and maintain the equipment. The
system seeks equilibrium—dynamic homeostasis. The good manager recognizes what can happen and adapts to the new situation.

B. Laboratory Subsystems

The management functions for a clinical chemistry laboratory are but
one segment of the universe of that laboratory. Bench functions are discussed elsewhere.

Certain managerial functions or systems are of importance to a manager
in clinical chemistry. Outside of the theoretical construct, to manage,
i.e., make decisions, one pragmatically must be concerned with at least
four areas: finances, personnel, information, and space. Each relates inextricably to the other.

Finances cover areas of budget preparation, purchasing, and financial
reimbursement. Personnel involves interviewing, hiring, and working
with people; evaluation of their competencies; and reward and discipline.
Information means the establishment of workloading recording, and the
interface of this data to the planning process.

Space subsumes everything as physical facilities impact upon the mission of organization. The wise use of present space and the good planning
of projected space is critical.

Space, people, money, and laboratory data are all interrelated and impact upon one another. Space is determined by workload, staffing, and money available.

Staffing is determined by amount of work, physical facilities, and money available to hire. Budget is dependent on workload documentation (data), which is a function of people and facilities. Each subset of activities are contingent upon the other and as we examine each as systems, they provide the grist with which to plan and make decisions. Each generate data of some sort. We live or die organizationally by our data—its availability and accuracy.

1. Financial System

It would be naive to discuss the management of an organization as complicated as a clinical laboratory without a discussion of the budgetary ramifications incumbent on any manager.

Financial management for a laboratory involves the generation of income and the establishment of a spending plan—the budget; this income–expenditure continuum involves the establishment of several record-keeping and accounting functions, including a *cost–accounting system* to establish fee schedules for billing and reimbursement from third parties. This implies an *accounts receivable system*. It involves a system of payroll and purchasing, which implies an *accounts payable system*. Each system means a set of books must be diligently kept for each type of transaction.

Generally speaking, laboratory directors use the systems already intact in the institutional setting for the establishment of budget, the expenditure of resources, and the acquisition of income. Occasionally, these tasks are decentralized.

A manager must be accountable for spending someone else's money. This is an awesome task, and must be faced with responsibility. This means the manager establishes a good workload recording system, perhaps computer generated, so as to provide the basis for cost accounting and budget justification, and maintains expenditure records to document expenses commensurate with workload. Billing procedures must also be well run and documented.

There are two categories of budgets in health care institutions—operating budgets and capital construction budgets. Capital construction budgets are generally long term over several years, and involve large pieces of equipment or buildings.

The operating budget is usually of most concern to managers. It represents planning—planning of resources and expenditures—and predicts income.

A budget is also a control device that delegates resources commensurate with delegated authority.

An operating budget can be expressed in several ways. A budget may be a global budget, the most flexible. With a global budget, a manager is given or allocated a fixed sum over a time by which he may spend any amount on personnel, equipment, or other expenses as he finds necessary to get the job done.

Less flexible and more common is the *line-item* budget which is a line by line statement of finances for specific allocations, e.g., each personnel position and/or each piece of equipment. It is understandable, but very frustrating to work with a line-item budget. It demands more planning and documents accountability.

The components of an operating budget differs with institutional environment, but generally includes the following categories.

a. Expenses
1. Salaries: (regular, parttime and vacation time students, residents, consultants, and, very importantly, fringe benefits).
2. Supplies: chemicals, reagents, glassware, expendibles (lab), expendibles (office), minor equipment, journals, etc.
3. Rent and leases: space and equipment, photocopying.
4. Interest on loans.
5. Utilities: telephone, light, heat, water, garbage disposal.
6. Service contracts: preventive maintenance, maintenance, general repairs, cleaning.
7. Professional expenses: dues for learned societies, licenses, travel, etc.
8. Insurance.
9. Research.
10. Teaching and training programs.
11. Equipment.
12. Overhead expenses: building amortization, share of nonincome producing department expense.

b. Estimated Revenues
1. Billing.
2. Third party payments.

Establishment of budgets, billing, purchasing, and cost accounting are usually functions of the institutional setting. A good laboratory manager learns "how they work and makes them work for him."

External to the institution is the source of income. Most of this comes from third party payers, such as private nonprofit Blue Cross/Blue Shield, private profit insurance carriers, and the government, through Medicare and Medicaid. The remainder is generated by the private pay patient. The rates of reimbursement are usually negotiated with the third parties based on workload and actual costs incurred in past delivery of service.

2. Personnel Management

Much of what professional managers practice in personnel matters is a human relations approach. Apart from the dynamics of how one interacts with subordinates or fellow team members, there are certain practical things that a laboratory manager must do in terms of personnel.

One of the most important things a manager can do is hire good people and let them do their jobs. The interview is, therefore, a critical point in personnel. A good manager must become skilled in interviewing prospective employees. Planning is important—understand what each position for which you are recruiting demands in terms of values and competencies. Review the applicant's credentials with these in mind. Do not fail to use references, and ask for references if none appear.

Plan your questions so as to elicit from the applicant the information you wish. When the interview is complete, write your evaluation per your predetermined standards, so as to make good comparisons of all candidates.

The good manager constantly evaluates the quality of the laboratory, which includes the staff. The yearly evaluation is an important part of the work relationship. All evaluations should be discussed with the employee, and put in writing as documentation, whether positive or negative, and placed in the employee's file. This performance appraisal becomes data for decision-making in regard to personnel matters.

Discipline, promotions, raises, all must be based on some rationale. Just as financial data is collected, so too should personnel information.

Management style determines the way in which a laboratory manager personally communicates his decisions, or, in fact, makes those decisions.

3. Management Information System

A laboratory has as its *raison d'etre,* information. Information exchange is the final output. The laboratory data that is provided for the clinician is his decision-making in patient care is also critical in evaluating the laboratory's capacity and capabilities. The laboratory manager can neither plan nor make those decisions that are critical in the continual process of making the laboratory responsive to the needs for better patient care without good data.

The laboratory organization can be described as a communications network in which information flow occurs. Information is critical in order to make decisions whether it is the decision to purchase a new piece of analytical equipment, establish a new determination, or promote a technologist. Information must be gathered, processed, and transmitted.

There is much evidence to make a case for laboratory computers, for the rush of test results mandate that an effective accurate system for test results be established. Budget does not always allow for a computer; however, whether manual or automated, the summary workload reports are the heart of an information network.

Managerially, a laboratory director must be accountable for funds that include personnel as well as equipment. He must justify budget and space, and he must have information for staffing decisions or future equipment purchases. One needs to know the quantity and quality of the product. Any change that is made (workload) must reflect in some management adjustment, and without an understanding of what is, the only process for decision-making is intuition, and that is not acceptable.

The management of this information system runs the gamut of a good manual system to a complex computerized system.

An accurate system for determining and monitoring the productivity of the work force of any organization is most obviously essential to enable that organization to be cost effective. The extreme emphasis being placed on the cost of health care delivery in recent times emphasizes the need of this constant monitoring of the productivity of these clinical laboratories. Every section of either hospital or "independent" based clinical laboratories will have to prove that it can be as cost effective as its counterpart in other laboratories or its very existence will be threatened. The clinical chemistry laboratory director can no longer be satisfied with only accurate, precise, and timely reporting of procedures in ways that satisfy the personal desires of the many clinicians being served. The cost of rapid data return, stat responses, redundant laboratory procedures, and excess quality control, will have to be determined, and those special services that are not cost effective, as well as clinically effective, will have to be given up or altered appropriately. Third party reimbursement agencies will most surely move in this direction.

Although various methods for workload recording have been used by many laboratorians for many years, the first successful attempts to develop a system that could be consistently used by most clinical laboratories was reported in Canada in 1970 (Canadian Schedule). The College of American Pathology subsequently developed a system that is quite similar to and is based on the above Canadian system (Laboratory Work-load). It is important to note that the development of a stable consistent system was most necessary to allow accurate and meaningful year-to-year comparisons. Obviously, the cost of each, or multiples of each, workload unit becomes a unit of comparison that all auditors and other health care administrators will find most interesting.

Although the details of these systems are too large in number and scope to describe here, several points deserve emphasis. The workload unit for both systems is cited as equivalent to 1 min of technical, clerical, and aide time. Unit values measure time for the following procedural steps: initial handling of the specimen, specimen testing, recording and reporting, daily or routine preparation, maintenance and repair, solution preparation, glassware wash-up, and technical supervision. They do not include speci-men collection. All quality controls, standards, and repeats are counted identically to the unknown specimens. Separate recording of them is appropriate. Specific definitions of these various items are provided.

Extensive and detailed study of the many procedures in use in clinical laboratories has yielded tables indicating the unit values (total minutes) needed to provide results for each procedure. Different values are pro-vided for individual methods and instrumental systems where appropri-ate. Official time-study formats are available for anyone wishing to de-termine the unit values for new procedures (Laboratory Workload, 1978).

Employment of such a uniformly accepted system produces at least several valuable parameters. Total workload, section by section, can be calculated by simply multiplying the total "raw count" for each proce-dure performed by its own unit value. Productivity (total workload/man-hours) for each section follows easily. Volume and cost of quality control becomes available, and should be noted carefully as one measure of the *quality* of a laboratory's performance. The value of these data become very apparent in justifying requests for both equipment and personnel.

Finally, careful and accurate collection of the raw counts for patient samples, standards, and control sera is essential to the process. Compu-terization of the process is almost essential in the larger laboratories. As laboratory personnel become involved in either manual or automated data collection systems, the importance of the data should be thoroughly ex-plained to all involved. Assignment of responsibility for the function in each section is essential.

4. Space Requirements

A steady expansion of workloads for clinical laboratories of 10–15% per year, although possibly now decreasing in rate, along with other changes in technology relevant to health care delivery, will probably continue to make many clinical chemistry laboratories obsolete. Clinical chemists should, then, prepare ahead of time for the responsibility and opportunity to plan for a new laboratory. They also should expect considerable opposition to their ideas from architects, engineers, and administrators whose thought processes are influenced by drastically different backgrounds and biases. For example, you may well recognize that the rapid pace of technological developments may invalidate some of your concepts by the time the new laboratory is ready for use. "They," however, may suspect you don't know your business when you first say so. Nonetheless, your plan must allow for remodeling at some near future date with the greatest of ease and least expense. Authorities at the Center for Disease Control in Atlanta have developed considerable expertise in such matters. Several excellent references are currently available and should be carefully studied (Baer, 1975 and Manual for Laboratory Planning and Design, 1973). These references will discuss the relationships of hospital population statistics to expected workloads and, therefore, to space requirements. A number of formulas for calculating space requirements from data on bed census, admissions per year, past workload records have thus been developed. However, constantly changing methodology, instrumentation and clinical utilization patterns make them useful only as guidelines in the planning and bargaining processes. Additionally, financial constraints and competition with other hospital functions may well limit the space allocated to the laboratory. However, one can always argue for the need of future expansion of laboratory space due to the ever increasing workload experienced in the past; and, therefore, argue for the geographical location of the laboratory that will allow the future expansion. Workload records are invaluable in projecting future space needs. The degree of centralization of clinical laboratory services also bears on space requirements.

The battle of centralized versus decentralized clinical laboratories will doubtless continue, at least in academia, because of the desire of many research-oriented clinicians to provide patient services directly and will thus affect clinical laboratory space requirements. The clinical chemistry director who inherits such a situation will soon observe at least the following two associated events: (a) the specialty laboratory wishes to provide service only on weekdays and (b) the clinician directing the specialty laboratory will leave for another position and the clinical laboratory will inherit the responsibilities overnight. Thus, centralization should be actively pursued in the planning process if success seems at all possible.

Finally, the following data on space requirements are included because the study was never formally reported in the literature. Amenta collected data from 28 clinical laboratory directors of medical school affiliated hospitals, which related each hospital population to the desired space requirements, for a report to the Academy of Clinical Laboratory Physicians and Scientists. He recommended several approaches (Amenta, 1974). For a hospital with service and research, one determines projected square footage by taking 30 net square feet per bed, and adding 12,000 net feet; or 0.8 net square feet per admission per year, plus 10,500 net square feet; or 0.45 net square feet per admission per year, plus 0.042 net square feet per outpatient visit per year, plus 8,250 net square feet. In each case, the additive square footage represents research space.

The actual design of the laboratory which obviously follows any space allocation, is much too complicated to discuss here. The above, and other references, should be consulted. Personal visits to other laboratories can be very valuable. A continuously updated file in such matters should become the property of any clinical chemist with the remotest chance of inheriting the problem.

As seen by each system, financial, personnel, space, and information, the data generated by each affect the other, and in so, support the other. The good laboratory manager understands this and uses this to his best use. The information flows from one network to the other, thus describing reality. Decision-making, the essence of a manager, must have information—the lifeblood of the enterprise.

IV. PLANNING AND DECISION-MAKING

A. Decision-Making Strategies and the Planning Process

Several theorists have provided models or techniques for decision making.

Kepner and Tregoe (1965), recommend that one analyze the what, where, when, and the extent of what is and is not, and look for the distinction or the change for guidance in decision making.

Blake and Mouton (1969), have developed a grid of leadership style around the extent to which a leader expresses a concern for people and a concern for productivity.

No single theory is all-inclusive, and can provide a recipe for leadership. Decisions in the laboratory, as well as other areas, are both long term and short term, and cover every aspect of the enterprise. A pragmatic approach can be recommended.

A decision is a leap of faith after all the analytical techniques have been used. Often we must make the leap, for our responsibility at times demands a decision—any decision.

Decision cuts across all aspects of the enterprise—organizational questions must be answered. Budgets must be prepared and decisions must be made regarding personnel, equipment, etc. It is expected that decision-making be based on a reason. The steps in reasoning are simple. Implementation is the illusive part of the process.

There are several steps.

1. *The analysis of the problem.* This is a statement of what is wrong or at least an identification of the issues. Some decision-makers suggest that a simple redefinition of the problem provides the simple solution. For example, the research and development people who designed the snap tab beer can revolutionized the industry. Their original problem was to design a better can opener; however, they redefined the problem not as a better can opener, but of an easier opened can. The analysis means one must obtain all the facts not unlike what the clinician does when he orders an SMA12 profile. It is a process of investigation of all the possible causes and identification of the real problem.
2. *The development of alternative solutions.* One turns to past experiences and/or the past experience of others to look for models to solve the problem. Creative managers brainstorm and develop alternate solutions to the problem. Administrative style determines this is an individual process or a team responsibility.
3. *The analysis of alternative solutions.* At this stage, the manager must weigh the advantages and disadvantages of each option. He plays out each scenario and often acts as the devil's advocate to aid in choosing the best alternative. It is important to note that one's alternatives may not all be good or bad, and one must determine which one maximizes one's gains and minimizes one's losses.
4. *The implementation of the decision.* Here the plan of action decided upon is put into action. Here is where the communication process begins.

It is sometimes difficult to operationalize these steps and separate them for they blur in what is a singular process.

There are several questions one can ask to facilitate the process:

1. What is the problem?
2. What are the pertinent facts?
3. Who should be involved in the decision?
4. How do the problems relate to the original objectives?
5. What are alternative solutions?
6. What do they cost?
7. For each alternative, what does this decision mean in the future?

8. What are the procedures for making it work?
9. How are the results to be tested?
10. What provisions are there for modification or change?
11. Is the decision-maker prepared to live with the results?

B. Laboratory Director as Leader

As the hospital and clinical laboratories grow in size and complexity, so do the educational and training requirements and the authority and responsibilities of the clinical chemist. The doctorate level clinical chemist in the academically affiliated medical center will have more influence on major policy decisions, e.g., selection of inhouse procedures, automation approaches, etc, than his or her counterpart at the smaller suburban or rural hospital. Similarly, the clinical chemist in the academic medical center will have greater opportunities to discuss the clinical significance of new and innovative techniques with clinicians. Both, however, will have to fight for resources needed to implement the policies established. Both will have to obtain the maximum productivity possible from the technical staff to enable the clinical chemistry laboratory to survive in today's highly competitive market. Both will have to help develop policies that result in the optimum combination of accurate, precise, and timely data production to assure support of clinicians for desired goals. Both, thus, will have to learn to become effective leaders.

To learn to lead effectively, each new supervisor or director will do well to seriously examine his or her own style of personal interactions with others in the light of the initial discussions in this chapter and in other discussions on personnel management (Bennington, 1978; Lundberg, 1975). A successful director must learn to direct without being too autocratic; to be respectful of other's needs and desires without trying to be one of the crew, to discipline and reward as objectively and fairly as possible, to delegate and monitor tasks and responsibilities, and to use lines of communication wisely and effectively.

The above statements obviously apply to any leadership role. There are, however, a number of leadership problems somewhat unique to laboratory medicine. Some of these are discussed as follows.

1. Communication with Hospital Administrators, Accountants, Auditors, and Government Executives and Legislators

You, as the Director, must learn to communicate effectively with the above types to be able to obtain adequate budgets, space, optimal legislation, etc. Yet, the gulf between you and "them" is enormous beyond description. The significance of monitoring therapeutic drug levels is not as obvious to administration as it is to you. Similarly, the purchase of a new multicolored framistan with automatic data reduction through interaction with dedicated digital computer assistance may well produce such attractive "trend analyses" reports of patient data that its purchase would seem to merit instant approval to you. But all that the accountant sees is the price tag and thus will quickly ask for the projected revenues. But, you say, this new approach may be somewhat more expensive, but the new data will decrease the time needed to diagnose "essential malignant stupidity." Administration may well ask any number of questions, e.g., how prevalent is the disease, or is this more important than new X-ray equipment? In short, you must learn to document your case in language familiar to the nonlaboratorian, to have your priorities established, and to have evidence of support of your clinicians for the project involved.

2. Communication with Clinicians

Clinicians have never, and probably never will have, received adequate training to assure optimum utilization of clinical laboratory services. They need help and often don't know it. You will probably have to convince them of the need of new procedures, etc. Get to know them in the lunchroom and attend the appropriate conferences. Find out what they want and via informal or formal discussions, explain what you need to do what they want. In the process, both you and the clinician will learn. This same clinician can well prove to be your best friend in your attempts to improve the quality of your services by taking your side in budget arguments with administration, who by and large do not understand why quality is often more important than cost.

3. Communication with Technical Staff

To assure the continuous delivery of clinically reliable data, a knowledgeable, conscientious, and dedicated staff of technologists is absolutely essential. You may direct, but they implement. The more understanding they have of the clinical significance of the data, the less will errors and delays occur. Productivity and accuracy go hand in hand with pride of performance. In-service training—both formal and informal—are essential to these goals. You must gain the respect of your technical staff.

Finally, the strategy and tactics to gain any goal should be carefully worked out. Lundberg (1975) in the section "Making Things Happen" provides a brief, but excellent, discussion of some of both.

V. IMPACT OF GOVERNMENT IN THE CLINICAL
    LABORATORY

Laboratory medicine does not exist in a vacuum, but rather is part of the total health care system, and must be responsive to external forces. The most significant external force, other than accrediting and licensing agencies, which impact upon the laboratory, is the Federal Government.

Two recent developments are the several attempts in recent years to pass federal legislation under the title "Clinical Laboratory Improvement Act, 1967" and the "National Health Planning and Resources Development Act of 1974." Both acts and subsequent regulations are still unfolding and will change forever the manner in which laboratories will do business.

The National Health Planning and Resources Development Act (PL 93-641) of 1974, has begun to change our way of thinking in health care delivery. The purpose of this legislation is to allocate resources for health care equitably throughout the nation; to establish minimal health care accessibility to all; to reduce excess expenditures; and hold the cost of health care down.

In 1965–1966, the federal government planted both feet into health care funding through Medicare and Medicaid. In 1974, the government, in reaction to huge opened expenditures to finance these programs, established the Health Systems Agencies (HSA), each representing a geographical region.

Governance of the HSAs are decentralized; however, certain guidelines must be adhered to in terms of representation. The legislation:

> authorizes the Secretary (*ed.,* of the Department of Health, Education, and Welfare) to enter into agreement with eligible entities for the designation of such entities as health systems agencies for health service areas established . . . as geographical regions appropriate for the effective planning and development of physical and mental health services. Each such health systems agency shall have as its primary responsibility the provision of effective health planning for its health service area and the promotion of the development within the area of health services manpower, and facilities which meet identified needs, reduce documented inefficiencies, and implement the health plans of the agency (Federal Register, 1975).

Government's role in health care planning, advisory at best in the past, will now be more controlled. "Planning" and "implementation" change the former relationship between the public and health care institutions of which the laboratory is a key part.

The decision-making powers of the Board of the HSA affects how one organizes health care for the region. Unlike the predecessors of Comprehensive Health Care Planning and the Regional Medical Programs, HSA has clout, with a 51–60% consumer representation.

Laboratories will directly be affected by HSA, namely for approval for new facilities and purchase of capital equipment. As health planning becomes more established, the HSA will have a larger role in all planning of future laboratory growth and effectiveness. If the technology can be obtained to do cost-effective laboratory work in bulk, then it may not be long before clinical laboratories are consolidated through direct action by local HSAs. Each year the HSA provides an Annual Implementative Plan that identifies special health care issues locally, and sets objectives and methodology to implement them.

The manager of a clinical chemistry laboratory must recognize the entrance of a new variable in the environment of health care, and be ready to deal with the results.

PL 93-641 has some stated and unstated assumptions:

1. Hospitals and other health care institutions, which undoubtedly cover the clinical chemistry laboratory, now are a "public interest" much like a public utility.
2. These institutions must be held accountable for operations and decisions effecting operations.
3. Decisions concerning the financing of health care and its delivery will no longer be made alone. Politicians, bureaucratics, professional planners, consumers, and practitioners will together make these decisions.
4. The Congress and the Administration view cost containment of health care as the overriding issue (Gottlieb, 1975).

As the impact of the Clinical Laboratory Improvement Act will be discussed in detail in Chapter 2, only one observation on it will be made here. In this observer's opinion (M.E.C.), that federal legislation permits the doctoral scientist (Ph.D.) to direct a clinical laboratory division adequately related to his/her scientific training is most important. Although some states, e.g., New York State, permit doctoral scientists to so do, legislation to the contrary has been proposed, e.g., in Texas in 1979.

REFERENCES

Amenta, Joseph, Report of the Academy of Clinical Laboratory Physicians and Scientists, 1975.

Report of the Academy of Clinical Laboratory Professionals & Scientists, 1974.

Baer, D. M. (1975). *Prog. Clin. Pathol.* **6,** 289–306.

Bennington, J. D., Böer, G. B., Louvau, G. E., and Westlake, G. E. (1977). "Management and Cost Control Tech- for the Clinical Laboratory." Univ. Park Press, Baltimore, Maryland.

Blake, Robert, R., and Mouton, J. S. (1969). "Building a Dynamic Corporation Through Grid Organization Development." Addison-Wesley, Reading, Massachusetts.

Canadian Schedule of Unit Values for Clinical Laboratory Procedures (1978). Statistics Canada, Health Division, Hospital Section, Ottawa.

Etzioni, Amitae (1964). "Modern Organization." Prentice-Hall, Englewood Cliffs, New Jersey.

Fanshel, S., and Bush, J. W. (1970). *Oper. Res.* **18,** 1021–1066.

Federal Register, Vol. 40, No. 202, Oct. 1975, 8803.

Gottlieb, S. R. (1975). "What Trustees Should Know About The Planning Law." pp. 12–14.

Gulich, L., and Urwich, L. (1933). "Papers on the Science of Administration." Institute of Public Administration, Columbia Univ. Press, New York.

Katz, D., and Kahn, R. L. (1966). "The Social Psychology of Modern Organizations." Wiley, New York.

Kepner, C. H., and Tregoe, B. B. (1965). "The Rational Manager: A Systematic Approach to Problem Solving and Decision Making." McGraw-Hill, New York.

Laboratory Workload Recording Method (1978). College of American Pathologists, 7400 North Skokie Blvd., Skokie, Illinois 60076.

Lundberg, G. D. (1975). "Managing the Patient-Focused Laboratory." Medical Economics Book Division, Oradell, New Jersey.

Manual for Laboratory Planning and Design (1974). College of American Pathologists. Chicago, Illinois.

McGregor, D. (1960). "The Human Side of Enterprises." McGraw-Hill, New York.

Odiorne, G. S. (1965). "Management by Objectives." Pitman, London.

Roethlesberger, F. J. and Dickson, W. J. (1939). "Management and the Worker." Harvard Univ. Press, Cambridge Massachusetts.

Simon, H. A., Smithbury, D. W., and Thompson, V. A. (1959). "Public Administration." Knopf, New York.

Taylor, F. W. (1911). "Scientific Management." Harper, New York.

The National Health Planning and Resources Development Act (PL 93-641) (1975). *Fed. Regist. No. 202,* **40,** 8803.

Weber, M. (1947). "The Theory of Social and Economic Organization." William Hodge, London.

Woodward, J. (1965). "Industrial Organization: Theory and Practice." Oxford Univ. Press, London and New York.

2

Laboratory Safety and Environmental Monitoring

WESLEY R. VAN PELT

I. INTRODUCTION

The purpose of this chapter is to provide the reader with the elements of safety as applied in a clinical chemistry laboratory. The more mundane safety and health practices such as the use of fire extinguishers and the safe handling of strong acids and bases are not discussed because (1) the

23

techniques are common to most laboratory and industrial workplaces and (2) common sense will usually lead the laboratory worker to the proper technique. Such general safety and health methodologies may be found in the regulations of the U.S. Occupational Safety and Health Administration (OSHA) and the many documents, studies, and recommendations of the National Institute of Occupational Safety and Health (NIOSH). Also, many texts are available on this subject (Manufacturing Chemists Association, 1972; Muir, 1977; Proctor and Hughes, 1978; Olishifski, 1979).

Therefore, this chapter will emphasize the safety problems which are specific to the clinical laboratory and which require the application of technologies not always easily available to the clinical laboratory technologist. In my opinion there are two such areas: radioactivity and infectious etiologic agents.

II. RADIOACTIVITY

A. Radiation and Radioactivity— An Historical Background

In the winter of 1895, a German physicist named Wilhelm K. Roentgen was experimenting with a partially evacuated glass "Crooks tube" through which he passed an electric current. He noticed that a nearby barium platinocyanide screen glowed when the electric current was turned on. The amazing thing was that the screen continued to fluoresce even when opaque material was placed between the tube and the screen. Roentgen called these mysterious rays "X rays" and had thus discovered radiation.

The news of Roentgen's discovery spread rapidly. Within a few months of Roentgen's first observation, physics laboratories throughout the world were turning their Crooks tubes into primitive X-ray tubes and taking crude radiographs of their hands and other objects using photographic plates.

This flurry of activity was not without its tragedy. It was soon learned that these new Roentgen rays could cause biological harm. A short exposure to the rays caused a reddening of the skin, or erythema. Longer exposure times caused burns and even death.

Another physicist, A. Henri Becquerel, heard of this discovery and set out to produce Roentgen rays by purely optical means using fluorescent chemicals. By February 1896, Becquerel had exposed a photographic plate through its opaque paper wrapping using crystals of fluorescent potassium uranyl sulfate. It soon became apparent to Becquerel that it was the element uranium that was the source of the X rays and the optical fluorescence was just a superfluous property. Thus, radioactivity was discovered by Becquerel only a few months after Roentgen first produced X radiation. In the next few years, Madame Curie and others discovered the natural radioactive elements radium, polonium, and thorium.

The years between Roentgen's discovery and World War II held a wide use of radiation for medical diagnosis and the treatment of disease. X rays were used for bone imaging and for the treatment of cancer. Radium became something of a health fad from about 1920 to 1940. Radium compresses and devices to infuse a glass of water with radon were used as a cure for various diseases. Thorotrast (containing thorium oxide) was used as a contrast medium for diagnostic radiograpy from about 1930 to 1945. Used for its opacity under X rays, the thorium was only incidentally radioactive. Many of these thorotrast patients developed radiation-induced tumors several decades after administered.

Radium was used as a component in luminous paint for watch and instrument dials. Many of the women who painted these dials with the radium paint subsequently developed bone cancer from internally deposited radium.

When the atomic age dawned in the mid-1940s, much was known about ionizing radiation and the biological damage it can cause. As a result of the early X-ray and radium experience, scientists were forearmed with the knowledge needed to protect the radiation workers of the new atomic age. The atomic energy industry has had a remarkably good record with respect to radiation accidents and fatalities. It is probably the only potentially hazardous industry in which safety developed along with the technology rather than after the technology had resulted in an unacceptable number of worker injuries and fatalities.

B. General Nature of Radioactivity

Many detection methods for immunoassay procedures have been developed, such as, particle agglutination, flocculation, immunodiffusion, fluorometry, etc. But the most sensitive, and presently most widely used technique, is radioimmunoassay in which the immunogenic molecule is tagged with one or more radioactive atoms, usually iodine-125 (^{125}I) or tritium (hydrogen-3, ^{3}H). The astounding detection sensitivity of the radioimmunoassay technique is evident when one realizes that one count from a nuclear detector results from the decay of *a single atom* attached to a single immunogenic molecule. A typical automatic gamma counter is capable of detecting with a confidence level greater than 99% less than 4 million atoms of ^{125}I assuming a 10-min counting time. For antigens of molecular weight 20,000 labeled with one ^{125}I atom each, this corresponds to a detection of 0.00013 nanograms.

Radioactivity refers to the ability of matter to undergo spontaneous nuclear disintegrations with a resulting release of kinetic energy and transformation of the atom into a different element. A radioactive disintegration (also called a decay or nuclear transformation) is accompanied by the emmission of *ionizing radiation* in the form of γ rays, X rays, β particles, α particles, energetic electrons, neutrons, etc.

This section outlines the properties and uses of radiation with emphasis on information most useful to the radioimmunoassay practitioner.

C. Iodine-125 and Iodine-131

Radioactive iodine has become the most useful radioactive species in the radioimmunoassay business. This is probably due to ready availability, convenient half-lives, and the ease of incorporation into biologically active organic molecules. The only two radioisotopes of iodine used in radioimmunoassay are iodine-125 (^{125}I) with a half-life of 60.1 days and iodine-131 (^{131}I) with a half-life of 8.05 days. And of these two, ^{125}I has achieved a clear advantage with its longer half-life.

Although ^{131}I has an inconviently short half-life (8.05 days), its concomitantly greater specific activity makes it useful when the sensitivity of the assay must be maximized. The half-life ($t_{1/2}$) and number of atoms (n) of any radionuclide are related by the equation:

$$A = n \ln 2/t_{1/2}$$

where A is the amount of radioactivity in disintegrations per unit time and ln 2 is the natural logarithm of 2(= 0.693). Thus, if the number of radioactive atoms is held constant, then the disintegration rate is inversely proportional to the half-life of the radioactive species. In this regard, a fixed number of ^{131}I atoms has a disintegration rate 8 times that of an equal number of ^{125}I atoms.

When an atom of ^{131}I decays, it emits a 0.61 MeV β particle (a high-speed electron) and a 0.36 MeV γ ray. In practice, it is almost always the 0.36 MeV γ ray which is detected and counted. The decay product (daughter atom) of ^{131}I disintegration is *xenon-131*.

^{125}I, on the other hand, decays by electron capture and emits a series of X rays, electrons, and a γ ray. Table I shows the primary ionizing radiations along with the abundance (average number per 100 disintegrations) of each type of emission. The photons (γ plus X rays) from ^{125}I are always detected and counted rather than the electrons. Even though the photon energy of ^{125}I is only about $\frac{1}{10}$ that of ^{131}I, they are both detected quite effi-

TABLE I

Photo Emissions from ^{125}I

Energy (keV)[a]	Intensity (%)[b]
27.2	39.8
27.5	74.2
31.0	25.8
35.5	6.7
total:	146.5%

[a] keV, kilo electronvolts (1 keV = 0.001 MeV).
[b] Intensity, percent photon abundance per disintegration (thus, on average, ^{125}I emits 1.46 photons for each atom which decays).

ciently in well designed gamma counters. In fact, ^{125}I has an advantage because of its higher photon abundance.

All radioactive materials, because of their ability to emit ionizing radiation, have an inherent degree of hazard associated with their use. The radioiodines have three particular characteristics that put them among the more hazardous radionuclides. First, iodine is a particularly volatile chemical, i.e., it tends to become a vapor. This makes containment of the material more difficult. Second, once it enters the body through inhalation, ingestion, or skin absorption, it concentrates and remains in the thyroid gland. About $\frac{1}{3}$ of the iodine taken into the normal human body is fixed in the thyroid gland where it "turns over" with a biological half-time of about 120 days. For ^{125}I, the radiological elimination rate ($t_{1/2}$ = 60 days) combines with the biological elimination rate ($t_{1/2}$ = 120 days) to produce an overall effective elimination rate with a half-time of 40 days. Thus, 30 microcuries (μCi) of ^{125}I accidentally taken into the body will result in about 5 μCi in the thyroid 40 days later.

The third hazardous characteristic of radioiodine is its ability to move through the ecological chain represented by atmosphere, grass, dairy cow, milk, human. Since this is a very efficient environmental pathway for radiation dose to man, the maximum permissible concentration (MPC) of radioiodines released to the general environment is much smaller than for many other radionuclides.

D. Tritium, Carbon-14, and Cobalt-57

Occasionally tritium (^{3}H) and even less often carbon-14 (^{14}C) and cobalt-57 (^{57}Co) are used as the radioactive isotope incorporated into the antibody.

Tritium and ^{14}C are both pure β emitters (i.e., no γ radiation or X rays) with β particle energies of 0.018 and 0.156 MeV, respectively. These are low or "weak" β energies and have a limited range in matter. For example, in unit density material such as water, the ranges of the tritium and ^{14}C β rays are, respectively, 0.0006 and 0.028 cm. Even in air, these weak β rays travel only 0.5 and 22 cm, respectively.

This range–energy relationship for tritium and ^{14}C has several important practical consequences for the laboratory. First, tritium and ^{14}C are hazardous only if taken into the body thereby producing internal irradiation. The dead layer of skin on the body is sufficient to absorb β radiation originating outside the body without damage to living cells. Second, film badge radiation dosimeters do not detect tritium or ^{14}C because the paper layer covering the photographic emulsion absorbs most if not all of the β energy without exposing the film. Thus, film badge dosimeters are ineffective in laboratories where the only radionuclides are tritium and ^{14}C. Third, tritium and ^{14}C must be assayed by liquid scintillation spectroscopy where the radioactivity and detector (scintillant) are intimately mixed. Fourth, tritium is not detectable at all with the usual hand-held portable radiation survey instruments such as Geiger counters. Carbon-14, however, is quite easily detected with a Geiger counter equipped with a Geiger tube with a thin (and fragile) end window.

Cobalt-57 is a radionuclide with a 267-day half-life. It decays by electron capture yielding a 0.12 MeV γ ray. The daughter atom is (nonradioactive) iron-57. Cobalt-57 is used predominantly in radioimmunoassay systems for vitamin B_{12} (cyanocobalamin), a molecule which contains an atom of cobalt.

E. Radiation Safety Program

How extensive must the administrative controls be for an effective radiation safety program in a clinical laboratory? It depends on the amount of radioactivity and frequency of use. It is convenient to imagine three levels, each of which requires a quantum jump in the extent of administrative control necessary. They are (1) the small general clinical laboratory, which may utilize a few commercial radioimmunoassay kits each week; (2) a large clinical laboratory employing many dozens of technicians who use a great many and variety of commercial radioimmunoassay kits each week; and (3) a large clinical laboratory which in addition labels its own antigens and/or antibodies with ^{125}I, ^{131}I, or tritium. Thus, the elements of a good safety program as discussed below should be adjusted to fit the size and extent of radiation usage.

The management of any sized clinical laboratory must appoint a single person who will have the responsibility for and the authority over the radiation safety program. This person, called the Radiation Safety Officer or Radiation Protection Officer, maintains all appropriate records and administers the program on a continuing basis.

In order to determine the location and quantities of all radioisotopes within the facility, a periodic *inventory* is performed, usually monthly or quarterly. The radioisotope inventory is useful in determining whether the laboratory's license limit for any particular radionuclide has been exceeded. For facilities with either general or specific radioisotope licenses, the inventory is a useful tool for monitoring the growth of radioisotope usage and planning for needed license ammendments.

A *radiation survey* should be performed routinely, perhaps monthly, by the Radiation Safety Officer or his designee. The survey consists of searching the work area for undiscovered contamination, excessive radiation levels, unsafe practices, improper equipment, etc. The surveyor uses a portable hand-held radiation survey meter and/or a box of small filter paper circles to wipe ("swipe," "smear") surfaces to pick up contamination. The filter paper circles are later analyzed for contamination levels, usually in disintegrations per minute (dpm) using either a gamma or liquid scintillation counter. Contamination above a predetermined level must be cleaned up by the person in charge of the contaminated item or area. An action level of 200 dpm per wipe is quite strict yet easily achievable in a facility with good handling and housekeeping techniques. A written record of these routine surveys should be maintained.

The portable radiation survey meter consists of a battery-operated electronic ratemeter which reads in counts per minute (cpm) and a detector or probe connected by a short electric cable. The ratemeter typically has 3 or 4 scale ranges covering zero to about 500,000 cpm. The probe best suited to a clinical laboratory is a thin sodium iodide scintillation detector because it is very sensitive to the low energy photon emissions from ^{125}I. Although an end window Geiger probe will detect ^{125}I photons, its detection efficiency is many times lower than that of the scintillation probe.

The use of radioactive materials must be restricted to authorized personel who have been trained in safe and proper handling techniques. This can be done informally in the smallest of laboratory operations, but should take on a more formalized structure in larger operations. For laboratories where several departments use radionuclides, the department supervisor should be made responsible for the radiological hygiene practices in that department. The Radiation Safety Officer should have control of the purchasing, receiving, storage, use, and disposal of radioactive materials in order to assure access by only properly trained and instructed personnel.

TABLE II

Activity Levels above Which Bioassay for ^{125}I or [131]I Is Necessary

| Types of operation | Activity handled at any one time in unsealed form making bioassay necessary[a] | |
	Volatile or dispersible[a] (mCi)	Bound to nonvolatile agent[a] (mCi)
Processes in open room or bench, with possible escape of iodine from process vessels	0.1	1
Processes with possible escape of iodine carried out within a fume hood of adequate design, face velocity, and performance reliability	1	10
Processes carried out within gloveboxes, ordinarily closed, but with possible release of iodine from process and occasional exposure to contaminated box and box leakage	10	100

[a] Quantities present may be considered the amount in process by a worker at one time. Quantities in the right-hand column may be used when it can be shown that activity in process is always chemically bound and processed in such a manner that ^{125}I or ^{131}I will remain in nonvolatile form and diluted to concentrations less than 0.1 μCi/mg of nonvolatile agent. Capsules (such as gelatin capsules given to patients for diagnostic tests) may be considered to contain the radioiodine in nonfree form, and bioassay would not be necessary unless a capsule were inadvertently opened (e.g., dropped and crushed). On the other hand, certain compounds where radioiodine is normally bound are known to release radioiodine when the material is in process, and the left-hand column may then be applicable. In those laboratories working only with ^{125}I in radioimmunassay (RIA) kits, the quantities of ^{125}I are very small and in less volatile forms; thus, bioassay requirements may be judged from the right-hand column.

Bioassay refers to a measurement made to assess the amount of uptake (internal contamination) of a radionuclide in a person. The only important bioassay technique in a clinical chemistry laboratory is the determination of the amount of ^{125}I bound in the thyroid glands of the radiation workers. The United States Nuclear Regulatory Commission has issued Regulatory Guide No. 8.20 (1978), which gives guidance on the need for and use of bioassay for licensees using ^{125}I and [131]I. Table II tells whether or not thyroid bioassay is needed at all. For laboratories using less than $\frac{1}{10}$ of the quantities shown in Table II at any one time, thyroid bioassay is not needed. For usage levels between $\frac{1}{10}$ and one times these quantities, professional judgment should be applied. If bioassays are not done at this level, a written evaluation should be kept on file and made available to U.S. Nuclear Regulatory Commission inspectors.

The thyroid bioassay technique involves placing a sensitive nuclear radiation detector close to the neck directly over the thyroid gland and accumulating counts due to the ^{125}I in the thyroid. Care must be taken to shield the detector from ^{125}I elsewhere in the room or on the subject's hands or clothing. The radiation background is taken with a neck phantom (solid plastic cylinder used to simulate the radiation absorption and scattering properties of a human neck) and subtracted from the patient count. The system is calibrated by placing a vial containing an accurately known quantity of ^{125}I in solution in a cavity in the neck phantom. The National Bureau of Standards sells an accurately calibrated ^{125}I solution that can be diluted (by weight or volume techniques) to make a suitable standard for calibrating the thyroid bioassay system. The calibrated ^{125}I solution is available for approximately $175 from the National Bureau of Standards.

A suitable radiation detector for the thyroid bioassay system is a thin sodium iodide scintillation crystal and integral photomultiplier tube. The optimal crystal is a flat cylinder about 2–3 mm high and about 50 mm across. Since the ^{125}I γ rays are almost completely absorbed in 3 mm of sodium iodide, thicker crystals do not increase the counting efficiency yet they have a higher background count rate and should, therefore, be avoided. The counting system should have an overall detection limit of about 0.003 μCi or less in the thyroid.

The interpretation of the quantity of ^{125}I in the thyroid is related to the Maximum Permissible Concentration (MPC) in air, which in turn is based on the maximum permissible radiation dose to the thyroid. The details and calculations relating these parameters, including elapsed times between intake and evaluation, are beyond the level of this presentation. However, United States Nuclear Regulatory Commission Regulatory Guide 8.20 (1978) recommends a hierarchy of actions which is reproduced in Table III as a guide.

In our experience, most personnel in a well-run clinical laboratory who continuously perform radioimmunoassays will have an equilibrium thyroid burden of less than 0.003 μCi of ^{125}I (the minimum detectable quality for our bioassay system). A few persons may have thyroid burdens in the 0.003–0.005 μCi range. Investigations leading to improvements in handling or storage techniques will often result in lowering the thyroid burdens of these individuals. On the other hand, persons who routinely label antigens with 1–20 μCi of ^{125}I will often reach an equilibrium thyroid level of 0.01 μCi or more, even with reasonably good techniques.

Environmental monitoring is required whenever greater than about 1

TABLE III

Action Levels for ^{125}I Thyroid Burdens

Level	Action
Thyroid burden exceeds 0.12 μCi	1. Investigate the operations to determine the cause of the exposure and to evaluate potential for further exposure. 2. If potential for further significant exposure exists, restrict the worker from further exposure until the situation is corrected. 3. Implement corrective action to eliminate or reduce the potential for further exposure. 4. Repeat the thyroid bioassay within 2 weeks to confirm presence of ^{125}I and estimate its effective half-life.
Thyroid burden exceeds 0.5 μCi	1. Carry out steps 1–4 above. 2. Refer the case to appropriate medical–health physics consultation for recommendations regarding therapeutic procedures that may be carried out to accelerate removal of radioactive iodine from the body. 3. Repeat the bioassay measurements at approximately 1-week intervals until the burden is at least below 0.12 μCi.

millicurie (mCi) of ^{125}I is used for labeling radioimmunoassay reagents. This is because it is difficult to meet the U.S. Nuclear Regulatory Commission limit of 8×10^{-11} μCi per cm^3 of air released to nonrestricted areas. Techniques such as high airflow hoods, closed reactions, keeping solutions (including waste) at a basic pH, and activiated carbon filtration of effluent air are all used to reduce environmental release concentrations. Sampling is done by drawing air through a small cartridge of activated charcoal at 1–10 liters/min and counting the charcoal in a well-type gamma scintillation counter.

F. General Laboratory Procedures with Radioisotopes

Laboratory handling and operating procedures for radioactive materials will vary with the particular radionuclide, the quantity, and the chemical form. However, the general rules presented below may be used as a general guideline for the safe handling of radioactive materials in the laboratory:

1. Disposable gloves and lab coat should be used whenever pipetting or otherwise dispensing radioactive solutions.
2. Never pipette radioactive solutions by mouth.
3. Absolutely no eating, drinking, smoking, or storing of food or beverages shall be permitted in radioisotope areas.
4. Disposable plastic-backed absorbent sheets should be placed on lab benches to absorb radioactive solutions.
5. A hand-held radiation survey meter should be used during and after all radioisotope operations to follow the progress of the radioactive species and to identify contamination. (Tritium cannot be monitored this way.)
6. Notify the Radiation Safety Officer of all spills, except those of a very minor nature.
7. All stored radioactive materials must be labeled with the radionuclide, the amount, and words "Caution—Radioactive Material," and the radiation caution symbol. When appropriate, include the user's name. Stored radioisotopes must be secure from unauthorized use.
8. No radioactive material should be put down the drain or otherwise enter the sewer. Place all radioactive waste materials in specifically marked waste cans or polyethylene jugs for disposal.
9. Radioisotope work should be done in the fume hood whenever the possibility of airborne contamination exists because of evaporation, flaking, dusting, or aerosolization of the activity.
10. A radiological clean-up should be performed after each major operation with radioactivity. All lab work areas, lab equipment, glassware, etc. should be decontaminated to near background levels.
11. Glassware should be thoroughly rinsed before dispatching to a central glasswashing facility. The first rinses should be disposed in the liquid radioactive waste container.
12. Never store food or beverages in refrigerators or freezers that also contain radioisotopes.

G. Waste Disposal

The disposal of radioactive waste material is regulated by the U.S. Nuclear Regulatory Commission or the various state agencies in the Agreement States. The state and federal regulations, however, are very similar, if not identical. General licensees, who may possess no more than 200 μCi of ^{125}I in units of 10 μCi each, have no restriction on their disposal methods. Thus, the most expedient disposal method is to flush liquid radioactive waste into the sewerage system and put solid waste into the ordinary trash. Care should be taken to remove or obliterate references to radioactivity such as the radiation caution symbol prior to disposal.

Laboratories with specific licenses must conform to Part 20 of Title 10 of the Code of Federal Regulations (or the equivalent Agreement State regulations), which, among other things, restricts the amounts and concentrations of radioactive material which can enter the sewer. Specific licensees must measure or calculate the radioactive concentration in the sewerage leaving their facility in order to assure compliance with these regulations. Solid waste generated by specific licensees is best given to a licensed waste disposal contractor for ultimate burial in a licensed low level radioactive waste landfill. Alternatively, solid waste containing ^{125}I can be held for 12–18 months for radioactive decay.

H. Licensing

All persons or institutions are required to be licensed in order to possess and use radioactive materials except for the case of license-exempt quantities, which for ^{125}I consists of single units less than 1 μCi each. Although a few radioimmunoassay kits are available that contain less than one microcurie, most are more and must be licensed.

General licenses are available to physicians, hospitals, and laboratories for *in vitro* clinical tests simply by filing a registration certificate with the United States Nuclear Regulatory Commission or Agreement State. (Except California, which is the only state where the general *in vitro* license is automatic without any registration required.) This general license allows the licensee up to 200 μCi of ^{125}I in units (kits) of 10 μCi each or less. A small clinical laboratory could comfortably operate under these quantity restrictions. However, expansion to a large variety of radioimmunoassays and/or to large test volumes might soon require the conversion to a specific license.

Specific licenses are tailored to the specific needs of a radioisotope program. It takes more effort and experience to obtain and administer a specific license than a general license. An applicant for a specific license must describe his proposed Radiation Safety Program, list all radiation detection instrumentation and describe the methods and frequency of calibration, list the people who will handle radioactivity along with their detailed training and experience, name a Radiation Protection Officer, describe the laboratory facilities (hood, benches, equipment, etc.), describe the waste disposal procedures, describe the personal dosimetry (e.g., film badge) method, and detail the bioassay procedure.

III. ETIOLOGIC AGENTS

A. Hepatitis

There are two types of hepatitis: type A hepatitis, which used to be referred to as infectious hepatitis, and type B hepatitis previously called serum hepatitis. Both diseases are viral in nature.

The symptoms of both types of viral hepatitis disease are similar in that they cause the same type of liver tissue abnormalities. These are tissue inflammation and destruction of the liver cells. The framework of the liver is not affected, and after recovery from the disease there is usually no permanent liver damage. Cirrhosis of the liver (an irreversible liver disease with fibrosis and nodule formation) resulting from viral hepatitis disease is extremely rare. Likewise, a hepatitis attack is not thought to increase the likelihood of future chronic liver disease.

Type A hepatitis has an incubation period of 15–40 days whereas type B hepatitis symptoms become evident only 50–160 days after exposure. After an attack, both types render the victim immune to future attacks of each disease. However, one type confers no immunity against infection from the opposite type. The symptoms of viral hepatitis include, weakness, jaundice, anorexia, headache, some fever, aches and pains.

In human populations, the type A hepatitis disease is spread by the fecal–oral route, often from close personal contact but also as a result of contaminated food or water. Type B, however, is transmitted primarily by direct injection into the victim's bloodstream, as with blood transfusions. Both diseases may be acquired by the clinical laboratory worker with the likelihood of infection being by accidental ingestion of type A virus contaminated material and accidental innoculation with type B virus contaminated material, as with inadvertent injection with a syringe needle. Recent information, however, has somewhat blurred these route distinctions, and laboratory workers can acquire either disease via either route, (Krugman and Giles, 1970).

There is clear evidence that clinical laboratory workers have a greater risk of contracting viral hepatitis than members of the general public. A questionaire survey was sent to members of the British Association of Clinical Pathologists regarding the circumstances of viral hepatitis attacks in clinical laboratories (Grist 1975; Grist 1976). The first survey report

covering the years 1970, 1971, and 1972, showed 5% of 244 clinical laboratories reporting one or more hepatitis cases in 1970, 7% of 215 in 1971, and
2% of 337 in 1972. A total of 36 laboratories reported 41 viral hepatitis
cases. This works out to an average annual attack rate of 111/100,000
clinical laboratory employees. Tests for hepatitis B antigen ("Australia
antigen") were positive for 17 cases, negative for 15 cases, and not done
for 9 cases, suggesting slightly more than one-half of the cases were type
B. None of the 41 cases were fatal and only 10 of the 41 required hospital
treatment. The report compares the clinical laboratory annual attack rate
to that of the general population of England, Wales, and Scotland of
27–51/100,000: about 2–4 times higher. The second report by Grist, covering 1973 and 1974 shows about the same overall picture with an annual
attack rate of 143 cases per 100,000 clinical laboratory employees.

A study measuring hepatitis B antigen (HBAg) and antibody (HBAb) in
the blood of hospital laboratory personnel in five Memphis, Tennessee
hospitals (Wruble et al., 1974) showed a clear pattern of positives when
compared with control groups consisting of clerical employees (none of
65) and employment applicants (5.5% of 200). Statistically significant pos-
itivity for HBAg or HBAb was found in 15% of 96 chemistry technicians,
14% of 43 pathologists, 13% of 85 hematology technicians, and 19% of 32
laboratory housekeepers. However, no increase over controls was seen
among hospital blood bank technicians (4% of 75). The fact that specific
laboratory technician groups had high hepatitis B while blood bank technicians were within the normal range suggested to the researchers that the
risk of occupational hepatitis can be controlled.

In a Scottish study, sera from 5071 inpatients was compared with that
from blood donors for HBAg and HBAb (Payne et al., 1974). The incidence of HBAg was similar in patients (0.116%) and donors (0.119%).
However, the incidence of HBAb was significantly higher in patients
(0.271%) than in blood donors (0.103%). Of the hospital inpatients, none
had a diagnosis of clinical hepatitis. The positive antigen or antibody
tests, therefore, indicated either a healthy carrier or a prior episode of hepatitis. This study indicates that greater than 0.1% of all blood specimens
sent to a clinical laboratory for routine diagnostic tests may be infected
with hepatitis. Thus, all specimens must be treated with great care, not
only the ones suspected of hepatitis contamination.

An editorial (British Medical Journal, 1976) discussed occupational hepatitis in British clinical laboratories and made the points: (1) hepatitis is
an occupational disease of clinical laboratory employees, but the number
of cases is small and the illness is relatively mild; (2) most occupationally
acquired cases are of the B type; (3) the risk of hepatitis comes from specimens from both hepatitis patients and from patients with no known evi-

dence of hepatitis; and (4) all specimens should be considered potentially infective.

B. Tuberculosis

Tuberculosis is a disease caused by several species of mycobacteria known as tubercle bacilli. Over 90% of all tuberculosis cases are pulmonary. The disease is spread by inhalation of the bacilli in aerosolized sputum from tuberculosis carriers. Treatment of tuberculosis consists of bed rest, good nutrition, and chemotherapy. Tuberculosis is an essentially curable disease due in large part to the drug isoniazid.

Clinical laboratory workers have an incidence of pulmonary tuberculosis that is 2 to 5 times that of the British general population (Harrington and Shannon, 1976). Tuberculosis is thus an occupationally acquired disease among laboratory workers and care must be taken by workers to avoid all contact with specimens contaminated with the tubercule bacillus.

Special precautions in handling tuberculosis specimens is given in several sources (Frankle *et al.* 1970; Collins *et al.* 1974; Central Pathology Committee, 1972). These precautions are based primarily on disinfection and sterilization of contaminated materials, ventilation control by working in a fume hood, avoidance of procedures that aerosolize the sample such as centrifugation and decanting, use of protective clothing such as gloves and coats, medical surveillance, and vaccination.

C. Immunization

The protective inoculation of laboratory workers provides a second line of defence against occupationally acquired infections—the first being the use of good safe technique. The decision whether to inoculate against a certain agent depends on (1) the expected frequency of the particular organism in the laboratory's samples; (2) the severity of the associated illness; and (3) the protective efficiency of the vaccine to be used.

Although each laboratory must assess its own risks and adopt a logical program for worker immunization, the British Public Health Laboratory Service has made some recommendations, which are summarized below (Collins *et al.*, 1974).

1. Live vaccines produce an immunity which persists far longer than killed vaccines and with a greater degree of protection. Laboratory workers can be exposed to far greater concentrations of an organism than the general public and as such may need a greater level of protection.

2. The Mantoux test should be given to all workers who handle tuberculosis specimens. Those with a negative reaction should be given
   BCG (bacille Caimette Guérin) inoculation. The Mantoux test
   should be repeated at least each 5 years because the reaction can
   revert to negative over a number of years.
3. Since smallpox has been successfully eradicated, there is no longer
   any need for this inoculation.
4. Inoculation for the typhoid bacillis should be offered to all laboratory workers and boosters given every 2 years.
5. Most laboratory workers will have had poliomyelitis immunity
   from childhood protective inoculations, but a booster dose should
   be considered.
6. Diphtheria is a rare disease and there appears to be no need for routine immunization of all laboratory workers.
7. Tetanus is not known to be acquired in the laboratory with any
   greater frequency than in the outside world. However, tetanus immunization is highly recommended for the population at large.
8. Occupationally associated rubella is thought to be rare. However,
   females working with rubella virus culture or serological tests
   should be tested for rubella antibodies and if not present, advised to
   be vaccinated.
9. Influenza virus also is not known to be laboratory acquired and
   there is no indication for routine vaccination of laboratory workers.
   The degree of protection from this vaccination is quite low.
10. Laboratory workers should be offered a screening test for serum
    hepatitis B surface antigen. The result will be useful in subsequent
    tests following accidental inoculation by a patient's blood sample.
11. Anthrax, plague, typhus, cholera, coccidiomycosis, and botulism
    are best considered on an individual basis. Where special proce-
    dures cause a greater risk from any of these, immunological sup-
    port should be considered as an adjunct to other safety practices.

D. Disinfection and Sterilization

Sterilization refers to the application of chemical agents or physical
conditions that are sufficient to kill all microorganisms. Disinfection is a
less than complete destruction of microorganisms, with the most resistant
forms surviving, albeit in reduced numbers.

Although there are many requirements for disinfection and sterilization
in the laboratory, perhaps the greatest challenge is the control of contamination by hepatitis B virus. This virus is more resistant to environmental
extremes than are many other viruses. Bond *et al.* (1977) report that hepa-

titis B virus has survived storage for 15 years at − 20°C, 6 months at room temperature, 4 hours at 40°C, exposure to ultraviolet light, triple ether extraction, β-propiolactone, benzalkonium chloride, and alcohol. However, boiling for 1 min readily inactivated the virus.

Bond *et al.* (1977) further report on much evidence that alcohol (ethanol and isopropanol) is ineffective in killing hepatitis B virus. Hypochlorite solution, on the other hand, at a concentration of 5000 ppm available chlorine, was sufficient to inactivate even undiluted hepatitis B surface antigen positive plasma.

Klein and Deforest (1963) studied the disinfectant properties of various chemical agents against both hydrophilic and lipophilic viruses. Sodium hypochlorite and iodophores were broadly effective with free chlorine or iodine concentrations down to 200 ppm being effective against all test viruses after 3–10 min contact time. Eight percent formaldehyde, 70–90% ethyl alcohol, and 2% glutaraldehyde were all effectively virucidal within short contact times. However, 95% isopropyl alcohol was not sufficient to kill to hydrophilic viruses. Likewise, phenol, phenol derivatives, and benzalkonium chloride were not uniformly effective disinfectants, with the hydrophilic viruses being the most resistant.

Much emphasis must be been placed on the physical cleaning of surfaces prior to the application of a chemical disinfectant. The removal of all visible contamination such as dried blood must be accomplished for effective disinfection.

Bond *et al.* (1977) after reviewing much of the hard data applicable to disinfection in the clinical laboratory put forth both "recommended" and "not recommended" chemical disinfectants. Those agents not recommended were done so because of insufficient sporicidal activity, the wrong properties for laboratory applications, or because they may be ineffective against hepatitis B virus.

Table IV summarizes Bonds's recommended and not-recommended disinfectants.

IV. SAFETY AND HEALTH ADMINISTRATION

A. Responsibility

The primary responsibility for safety lies with the laboratory worker, his or her supervisor, and the entire organizational up to the top management position within the corporation or institution. The adage that "safety is everybody's responsibility" has taken on additional impact in recent years with respect to the legal liability for occupational accidents.

TABLE IV

Recommended and Not-Recommended Disinfectants for the Clinical Laboratory

Recommended	Not recommended
Ethylene oxide gas ($3\frac{1}{2}$–16 hours)	Ethanol and isopropanol
Formalin (8% formaldehyde, aqueous)	Iodine
Formalin (20% in 70% alcohol)	Phenol and phenolics
Alkalinized glutaraldehyde, 2%	Quarternary ammonium compounds
Sodium hypochlorite (500–5000 ppm available chlorine)	Hexachlorophene
Iodophors (500–5000 ppm available iodine)	Mercurials

Responsibility for correcting unsafe conditions rests with the highest level manager who knows or should know about the condition.

An effective way of emphasizing the proper relationship of job safety and job performance is to include responsibility for safety in the written job descriptions for all appropriate line positions. Then, during the formal performance review of each employee, his or her safety performance can be discussed and areas for improvement can be targeted. Also, in this way, safety performance can be tied directly to annual salary or wage increases.

Another effective technique is to incorporate safety-related procedures and precautions into the laboratory's standard operating procedures and operating instructions. Thus, the written instructions for an analytical procedure will emphasize not only steps to get the correct answer but steps to minimize personal risk and environmental impact.

B. The Safety Committee

Probably the most effective tool management can use to improve the safety performance of an organization is an active, functioning, and aggressive safety committee.

The first thing a safety committee needs is a charter or mandate from top management and its continued support. Without this important backing, even the most well-meaning safety committee will soon become frustrated and ineffective. The committee should be composed of front-line workers (i.e., lab technicians), supervisors, managers, and administrators. This broad cross section of jobs assures that the committee is aware of the problems and needs of the laboratory workers and has the authority to commit funds and make changes whenever required to improve safety.

The committee should constantly review the state of safety within the organization. This is accomplished by reviewing all accidents, near-accidents, occupational illnesses, spills, fires, etc., and institute steps to prevent future occurrences. Another technique is the formal safety inspection carried out by all or part of the committee.

It is imperative that the committee have a chairperson, have regular meetings (monthly is suggested), keep written minutes of all meetings and inspections, follow up on all recommendations, and keep management informed of all activities of the committee.

REFERENCES

Bond, W. W., Peterson, N. J., and Favero, M. S. (1977). *Health Lab. Sci.* **14,** 235–252.

British Medical Journal (editorial) (1976). *Br. Med. J.,* p. 778.

Central Pathology Committee (1972). "Safety in Pathology Laboratories." Department of Health and Social Security, London.

Collins, C. H., Hartley, E. G., and Pilsworth, R. (1974). "The Prevention of Laboratory Acquired Infection." HM Stationery Office, London.

Frankle, S., Reitman, S., and Sonnenwirth, A. C. (1970). "Gradwohl's Clinical Laboratory Methods and Diagnosis," Vol. 2, 7th Ed., pp. 1267–1268. Mosby, St. Louis, Missouri.

Grist, N. R. (1975). *J. Clin. Pathol.* **28,** 255–259.

Grist, N. R. (1976). *J. Clin. Pathol.* **29,** 480–483.

Harrington, J. M., and Shannon, H. S. (1976). *Br. Med. J.* **1,** 759.

Klein, M., and Deforest, A. (1963). *Soap Chem. Spec.* **39,** 70–72.

Krugman, S., and Giles, J. P. (1970). *J. Am. Med. Assoc.* **212,** 1019.

Manufacturing Chemists Association (1972). "Guide for Safety in the Chemical Laboratory." Van Nostrand-Reinhold, Princeton, New Jersey.

Muir, G. D. (1977). "Hazards in the Chemical Laboratory," Chem. Soc. London.

Olishifski, J. B. (1979). "Fundamentals of Industrial Hygiene," 2nd Ed., Nat. Safety Council, Chicago.

Payne, R. W., Barr, A., and Wallace, J. (1974). *J. Clin. Pathol.* **27,** 125–129.

Proctor, N. H., and Hughes, J. P. (1978). "Chemical Hazards of the Workplace." Lippincott, Philadelphia, Pennsylvania.

U.S. Nuclear Regulatory Commission (1978). "Applications of Bioassay for I-125 and I-131." Nuclear Regulatory Commission, Washington.

Wruble, L. D., Masi, A., Levinson, M., Rightsell, G., Bale, P., and Bertram, P. (1974). *Gastroenterology* **66,** 800.

Criteria for Kit Selection in Clinical Chemistry

JAMES E. LOGAN

I. INTRODUCTION

A. General

The continuing increase in production and use of reagent kits for determining constituents in body fluids has made it essential to define criteria for kit selection in clinical chemistry. In 1972 the Center for Disease Control, Atlanta, compiled a list of test kits available for use in clinical laboratories. Barnett (1977), in his review, indicated that 1257 of these were designed for clinical chemistry. Logan and Taada (1977) found as a result of

CLINICAL BIOCHEMISTRY
Contemporary Theories and Techniques, Vol. 1

a survey in Canada in 1975 that at least one kit was being used for clinical chemistry in 640 hospital laboratories out of a total of 819 surveyed. There was also evidence even at that time of the growing popularity of radioimmunoassay (RIA) kits. According to the 4th RIA directory published by Sweeny (1978), 60 different companies were producing approximately 440 products in kit form for radioimmunoassay. Brown (1976) reported in a 1975 College of American Pathologists' (CAP) survey that 3162 out of 6614 laboratories, i.e., 48% used kits for the analysis of at least one of the six constituents surveyed. There was a clear trend in that survey for kits to be used more frequently in smaller hospitals. Sixty-eight percent of laboratories in hospitals under 50 beds used kits, whereas in hospitals from 301 to 500 beds the number was only 24%. Kits were used least often for bilirubin analyses, i.e., 29%, and most often for cholesterol, i.e., 39% of survey participants.

Broughton (1978) attributes the proliferation of kits on the market to laboratory directors seeking to set up simple tests at minimum capital cost. He points out that there are very few guidelines available on how to select a method for routine use and that no matter how well documented the procedure may be it must be evaluated in the user's laboratory. Laboratories of varying sizes and in different locations have quite different requirements for the use of kits. The accuracy and the precision which is needed in order to meet the clinical criteria may vary somewhat but it is the intent in this chapter to examine the basic criteria required to select those products which are suitable for use in the clinical chemistry laboratory. Articles have appeared in the literature dealing with evaluation of kits in which different approaches have been recommended for carrying out these kinds of assessments. See, for example, Barnett (1965, 1972), Barnett and Youden (1970), Büttner et al (1979b), Westgard et al. (1976, 1978a,b,c,d), Witherspoon (1976), Kim and Logan (1978a,b), Lloyd (1978), Neilsen and Ash (1978), and Rubin et al. (1979a,b). Selection of a kit for use in the laboratory cannot be properly made in the absence of an evaluation process to determine whether the selection made was the correct one. The published evaluation procedures will be reviewed and from this process a recommended set of criteria for kit selection will be presented.

Kits were first introduced on the North American market about 1956. They are now available to laboratories all over the world and their reliability has become a source of concern to the World Health Organization (WHO). The Expert Panel on the Evaluation of Diagnostic Reagent Sets of the International Federation of Clinical Chemistry (IFCC) with WHO support has drafted provisional recommendations in the form of guidelines for the evaluation of clinical chemistry kits (Rubin et al., 1979a,b), and Logan et al. 1981a,b). These guidelines will be used primarily by developing countries to screen products that are being offered for sale to their laboratories.

B. Definitions

A kit is defined by Rubin *et al.* (1979a) as "two or more different clinical or general laboratory materials (excluding reconstituting materials), with or without other components packaged together and designed for the performance of a procedure for which directions are supplied with the package." Other terminology used throughout this chapter adheres to that published by the IFCC Expert Panel on Nomenclature and Principles of Quality Control in Clinical Chemistry (Büttner *et al.*, 1979a,b). The above kit definition is the one used in this chapter. There are other definitions of kits or *in vitro* diagnostic products that are much broader in nature, e.g., the one published in the Federal Register (Edwards, 1973), which defines *in vitro* diagnostic products as those reagents, instruments, and systems intended for use in the diagnosis of disease or in the determination of the state of health in order to cure, mitigate, treat, or prevent disease or its sequelae. Many of the kits produced are designed to be used with a particular instrument system, but for the purposes of this discussion no attempt will be made to consider the merits of instrument systems. Evaluations of systems that incorporate the use of reagent kits have appeared from time to time in the literature. See, for example, Logan and Sunderland (1970), Sunderland and Logan (1971), Crowley and Alton (1971), Loeb and Bauman (1971), Sunderland *et al.* (1972). Carey *et al.* 1974), Chong-Kit and McLaughlin (1974), Henry and Saunders (1975), Passey *et al.* (1975), Chua and Tan (1976), Haeckel (1976), Bostick and Mrochek (1977), Fingerhut (1978), Ijpma *et al.* (1978), Lam and Tan (1978), Pearson (1978), and Porter and Roberts (1978). In addition to these examples, "Instrument Reports" have appeared for several years as a monthly feature in *Lab World,* and the American Clinical Consumer Institute also publishes a monthly report entitled "The Clinical Consumer Report," which gives reports of evaluation of kits and instruments.

C. Kits versus Other Clinical Chemistry Methods

A number of reasons may be cited why kits are used in clinical chemistry laboratories instead of the more classical manual or automated procedures. They may often be purchased for use in addition to the routine methods, e.g., in stat and night testing. Kits are particularly attractive for use in those laboratories where either the workload or the capital budget is insufficient to warrant automation. Their use avoids outlay of capital whereas ready-made reagents provided together with generally simple procedures reduce the time a technologist requires to carry out a test. In very small laboratories where the personnel may not be adequately trained in reagent preparation or in setting up new methods, reliable kits can play an important role. In larger laboratories they may be also attractive where personnel are too busy to spend time in reagent preparation. In a physician's office or clinic, kits can be useful to provide rapid information without the need for referral to an outside laboratory. In all such situations, one should be able to obtain with the kit results of equivalent accuracy and precision to those of the more classical procedure. Criteria are necessary to select those kits capable of meeting this requirement. It is outside the scope of this chapter to consider if a kit should or should not be used instead of a manual or automated procedure in any given situation.

D. Types of Kits

The categorization of kits can be made in a manner similar to that used to categorize analytical methods in clinical chemistry, e.g., chemical methods in which an endpoint reaction is used to measure the constituent quantitatively following color formation. There are other chemical methods in which an enzyme is used in a reaction to measure nonenzyme constituents kinetically, e.g., glucose. In others, a kinetic reaction is used to measure the enzyme activity where the constituent itself is an enzyme. More recently, RIA and competitive protein binding (CPB) kits have been developed to measure in nanogram amounts those hormones, proteins, protein-bound compounds, antigens, and drugs that circulate in the blood. Enzyme-linked assays are also being produced in kit form in which the ligand is bound to enzyme rather than to a radioisotope so that enzyme activity measurement is used to monitor the level of the constituent being assayed. These kits thus avoid the hazard to the technologist in handling radioactive reagents, but at the same time these generally lack the sensitivity of the RIA tests. Despite growing popularity of RIA kits, their precision is still somewhat unsatisfactory and care must be taken in making a selection from among RIA products.

II. REVIEW OF PUBLISHED CRITERIA

A. Labeling and Enclosed Literature

One of the criteria which must be considered in the selection of a kit is the adequacy of the labeling and enclosed literature provided by the kit manufacturer. In the early years of kit development before any government regulations existed to control these products, the labeling and the literature provided for the users' instruction were often woefully inadequate and sometimes misleading. This situation has improved due to regulatory processes, and it is now possible to make reasonable decisions on the suitability of a kit for a given testing application from a review of the enclosed literature. The first attempt to correct this fault was made in 1965 by the Committee on Standards and Controls of the American Association for Clinical Chemistry, which drafted a policy regarding reagent sets and kits. This policy contained a number of recommendations indicating the type of information the distributor or kit manufacturer should make available to the prospective purchaser or user (AACC Committee, 1966). Krynski and Logan (1968) prepared an arbitrary scoring procedure based on 15 points covered in these recommendations and subsequently used this system for rating the literature in a series of evaluation of kits (Logan, 1972). This procedure was more recently expanded to cover 20 points and includes requirements contained in North American governmental regulations (Kim and Logan, 1978a). The National Committee for Clinical Laboratory Standards (NCCLS) also produced a voluntary consensus standard based on the labeling of laboratory reagents (NCCLS, 1975). Some improvement in labeling and enclosed literature resulted from the influence of these professional organizations on kit manufacturers and by the publication of results of kit evaluation which showed comparative data for different manufacturers. It was, however, only by passing of legislation making it mandatory that certain information be provided to the user that marked improvement has been noted.

The labeling requirements for *in vitro* diagnostic products for human use were published in the Federal Register (Edwards, 1973). In Canada regulations respecting medical devices, which include *in vitro* diagnostic kits, were published containing the requirements for labeling of these products (Medical Devices Regulations, 1975). The U.S. regulations list nine sets of information that must appear on the label and a further 15 items that should be contained in the package insert. These requirements enable the user to properly identify the product, its lot number, its manufacturer and distributor, the composition of its reagents, its expiration date, and its intended use. Also provided therein are the necessary precautions for its handling, storage, directions for use, expected performance based on actual field testing, information on its test capacity relative to cost, and its compatibility with commonly used laboratory instruments. The principles of the test are given and pertinent literature references on which it is based so that the technologist may become fully informed about the test. The availability of kits on a worldwide basis has caused WHO to be concerned that inferior quality diagnostic reagents might be sold to laboratories in developing countries. As a result, the IFCC Expert Group on Diagnostic Reagents and Kits was asked to prepare a document for the labeling of clinical laboratory materials for use, particularly in these countries. This document has now been prepared as Part I of a provisional recommendation on evaluation of diagnostic kits (Rubin *et al.* 1979a). The author has prepared a score sheet based on these labeling recommendations for use as a subsequent part of the same provisional recommendations (Logan *et al.*, 1981a).

B. Performance Requirements by Regulatory Bodies

The evaluation of performance of a diagnostic kit by a governmental regulatory body often differs in its approach from that of the clinical laboratory scientist. The former is interested to know if the performance of the kit meets the manufacturer's claims whereas the latter wishes to know if it is capable of producing results of sufficient accuracy and precision so as to be meaningful to the physician in making a diagnosis or in monitoring a course of therapy. The claims of the manufacturer for his product may or may not be related to the clinical needs. In Canada, under medical devices regulations, the manufacturer of an *in vitro* diagnostic device is required to provide information on its performance characteristics. These, in turn, are defined as the properties and qualities of the device associated with its capacity to carry out its patient-related functions. The manufacturer will be required to submit detailed information on all parameters likely to affect the performance characteristics (e.g., time, temperature, pressure, pH, ionic strength, serum matrix effects, blanks, reagent concentrations, special additives, interfering substances, etc.). The description of each performance characteristic must have associated with it a quantitative statement of its precision and accuracy as well as its reliability if these are related to the capacity of the device to fulfill its claims and patient-related functions. For example, the manufacturer of a kit for glucose determinations would be required to submit quantitative information such as within-day and day-to-day precision, accuracy, sensitivity, test and linearity ranges, interferences, expected range, etc. The product then would be assessed in relation to whether it performs analytically according to the claims set out by the manufacturer. The laboratory scientist is still left to judge if these claims are acceptable for use in the clinical setting in which the kit is to be used.

Originally the United States Regulations in respect of performance differed in that the performance of the kit was to be matched against that of a product class standard, i.e., a reference procedure generally accepted to yield results that would be clinically useful. A product class standard for measurement of glucose in serum or plasma was under development when the Medical Devices Amendment was introduced in 1976. This amendment covers the regulation of *in vitro* diagnostic products and its implementation has delayed, for the present, further development of product class standards. Specifications for standards to be used in the evaluation of kits are now being developed with the assistance of the Center for Disease Control (CDC) and the cooperation of NCCLS. Particular attention has been directed toward some subgroups of kits, e.g., RIA tests for digoxin. NCCLS (1976) has developed guidelines for ligand assays. Reference methods and pool material for digoxin have been prepared by CDC and NCCLS. The criteria for judging the acceptability of labeling of *in vitro* diagnostic products in the United States are those mentioned above (see Section II, A).

C. Performance in Relation to Clinical Requirements

The most important criteria in the selection of a kit in the clinical chemistry laboratory are those directed toward identifying the product that will perform the best in relation to the clinical requirements of the test. Even if the protocol and methodological aspects are favorable to the use of the kit, the kit will not be acceptable if it does not perform sufficiently reliably at key medical decision levels for the physician to use in making a diagnosis or in monitoring treatment of the patient.

There are a number of steps in the process of making the selection of a kit and ensuring that the selection has been the right one. These will be considered under a number of subheadings and the literature discussing these topics will be reviewed. The steps may be considered as follows:

1. Definition of the requirements of the method
   a. Practicability characteristics
   b. Methodology characteristics
   c. Performance characteristics
2. Technical literature search and kit selection
3. Kit evaluation
   a. Evaluation of precision
   b. Evaluation of accuracy
   c. Evaluation of specificity
   d. Evaluation of sensitivity
   e. Statistical approaches for evaluation of data
   f. Performance standards
   g. Criteria for judging acceptability

1. Definition of the Requirements of the Method

Westgard (1978a) points out that first in the process of selection of a clinical chemistry method a careful definition of the requirements of the method is essential. This applies equally to the selection of a kit since it is necessary to select from the commercial sources available that kit which will most likely fulfill the laboratory's requirement for a method. These requirements should be set down before the kit selection process begins and should include the practicability, methodology, and performance characteristics of the kit.

a. Practicability Characteristics. Several authors have listed a number of factors, which may be called practicability characteristics. See Carey *et al.* (1974), Büttner *et al.* (1979b), Barnett (1977), Broughton (1978), Neilsen and Ash (1978), Rubin *et al.* (1979b), and Westgard *et al.* (1978a). Broughton (1978) has listed five factors, which may be considered under this title and about which little factual information appears when most analytical methods are published in the literature. These are speed, cost, skill requirements, dependability, and safety. Barnett (1977) names speed, convenience and cost as factors to be considered secondary to the adequate performance of a kit. Westgard (1978a) uses the term *application characteristics* and defines these as factors that determine whether a method can be implemented in a particular laboratory. He lists under these cost per test, types of specimens, sample volume, turnaround time, rate of analysis, workload, run size, equipment and personnel requirements, and safety considerations. Neilsen and Ash (1978) have published a protocol for the adoption of analytical methods in the clinical chemistry laboratory and list 19 points for examination before considering using a method for patient care in service laboratory. They point out that the need for the test must be established as it would be impractical to set it up unless it provides relevant and useful information to the physician. They have not categorized certain points as practicability characteristics, but they do mention that requirements for sample size, speed of analysis, personnel and training, equipment and reagents, assay conditions, and cost of the test should be considered. Büttner *et al.* (1979b) drafted recommendations for IFCC on the assessment of analytical methods for routine use that also list speed, cost, technical requirements, dependability, and safety as factors related to the practicability of a method. They point out that for technical skill requirements and safety it may be difficult to obtain objective data, but they consider subjective opinions useful provided they are identified as such. Data on dependability can only be acquired from long-term use in a number of laboratories. Rubin *et al.* (1979b) have prepared for the IFCC a list of practicability characteristics for use in selecting kit methods which consider type and volume of specimen, operating requirements, service requirements, consumables requirements, technical skill and training, safety problems, and equipment maintenance.

b. Methodology Characteristics. *Methodology characteristics* are defined by Westgard (1978a) as those factors, which, in principle, should contribute to the best performance and which are concerned with chemical sensitivity and chemical specificity. It would seem, therefore, that these latter two factors might also be considered in what Westgard separately calls performance characteristics and which include precision, recovery, interference, accuracy, and sometimes detection limit. The IFCC Committee on Standards (Büttner *et al.* 1979b; Rubin *et al.* 1979b) in their recommendations uses the term reliability characteristics to encompass not only sensitivity and specificity but also accuracy and precision. When considering the suitability of a kit, the relevant data on these characteristics as provided by the manufacturer or given in the literature references must be examined and then confirmed by evaluation of the product in the laboratory. Neilsen and Ash (1978) indicate that a method must be selected that has sufficient sensitivity to detect accurately those concentrations of analytes both below and well above the normal range of values without requiring sample dilution or causing any significant carryover to the other samples within the run. They stress that the method must be specific for the analyte so that the results will not be significantly influenced by other common sample or reagent constituents. The wavelength chosen for measurement should be one that yields maximum absorbance of the assay product with a minimum absorbance due to nonspecific chromogens. Büttner *et al.* (1979b) state that assessment of specificity is open-ended, because one must regard any food or drug as a possible interfering material until proven otherwise. Thus, the specificity of the method will depend on the type of specimen analyzed. The known limitations of specificity in a method should be given in the description of the method (or kit instructions) as very few analytical methods in clinical chemistry are completely specific for one analyte and free from interference from all the components that may be present in a patient's specimen. Büttner *et al.* (1979b) relate the chemical sensitivity of a method to the amount of analyte required to give a meaningful result so that the greater the sensitivity of the method, the smaller will be the amount of analyte required for detection. This same committee (Büttner *et al.*, 1979a) has defined detection limit as the smallest single result which, with a stated probability (commonly 95%), can be distinguished from a suitable blank. The method or kit chosen then must possess sufficient sensitivity to detect the analyte at those concentrations that have medical significance. The definition of Galen and Gambino (1975) for specificity and sensitivity of a test should not be confused with those used here. These authors refer to the capacity of a test to characterize, respectively, the incidence of true-negative results in disease-free subjects and the incidence of true-positive results in subjects known to have the disease. This is a case of relating the test directly to the presence or absence of disease rather than to the chemical detection of the analyte.

c. Performance Characteristics. Westgard *et al.* (1978a) defines performance characteristics as those factors which, in practice, demonstrate how well the method (or kit) performs. In the selection of a kit, information should be available or should be experimentally obtained to establish its analytical or linear range, precision, accuracy, detection limit, susceptibility to interference, and its performance in the recovery of added analyte. The requirements for performance of these factors should be determined in relation to the clinical requirements of the test. It is necessary to know the types of patients for whom the kit procedure is to be used, the range of concentrations expected, the workload, the demands on turnaround time, precision, accuracy, etc. Information of this kind may be found in the literature and by consultations with physicians requiring the test.

The large-scale proficiency testing programs in which many clinical chemistry laboratories now participate are generating data that provide information on the performance of diagnostic kits. Brown (1976) published data that showed the results achieved by kits for six constituents in 3162 institutions in the College of American Pathologists' (CAP) survey program. The agreement among results obtained by kit users was found to parallel that achieved by users of manual methods. Brown has pointed out that the generation of data of these kind from large-scale surveys could become a powerful force in kit selection. The limitations of such data in assessing kit performance were discussed by him and are summarized as follows:

1. Most survey specimens contain constituents with concentrations either in or close to the normal range so that good performance may not mean that the kit is equally capable of good precision and accuracy in the abnormal range.
2. Little information will be obtained concerning specificity in the presence of interfering substances as found in patient specimens since survey specimens usually contained few of these.
3. Incorrect categorization of the methods by participants can contribute to erroneous information concerning kit performance.
4. The modification of a kit by a manufacturer between the time the survey results were obtained and the data published could easily be missed. On the other hand, we believe that such data could provide useful information for kit selection if consistently poor survey results were associated with a particular manufacturer's product. The opposite is, however, not necessarily a reliable indication of a kit's

good performance since survey specimens are frequently given more than routine attention.

Barnett (1971) suggests that it is well to accept the advice of respected laboratories in selecting a kit, but at the same time points out the weakness that the other laboratory may not have used the kit in exactly the same way. Depending on the laboratory, it is possible that the clinical requirements for performance of the test may not be the same. At the time of publication of Barnett's statement, certain products bore the CAP seal, which indicated that performance claims had been verified by an independent evaluator selected by the CAP. This type of certification did not prove very popular among manufacturers, probably due to cost and delays in production. Thus, to seek a CAP certified product as a requirement would eliminate many good ones that had not been tested in this way. Kits should be selected which show minimal lot-to-lot variation in performance but one can really only check on this through proper internal quality control procedures. Broughton (1978) states that when an analyst is considering the suitability of a method (or kit) he must obtain information about the reliability characteristics, i.e., precision, accuracy, specificity, and sensitivity, and preferably in the form of quantitative data so that judgments can be made objectively. He indicates that these four characteristics are the primary ones and other factors such as stability, carryover, linearity, etc., which may be separately quantified in performance assessments are all contained in the primary ones. The IFCC Committee on Standards (Büttner *et al.*, 1979b; Rubin *et al.*, 1979b) also recommends that numerical data be obtained for reliability characteristics so that the analyst can select a method (or kit) that will meet his required standards of performance which, in turn, will depend on the purpose for which the method is used.

2. Technical Literature Search and Kit Selection

When one has carefully defined the application and reliability characteristics of a kit required in a particular laboratory, the next step is to search the technical literature to find what kits employ the method best suited for the test. This may be done by consulting the advertiser's literature, e.g., publication of kit directories appear from time to time such as the 4th RIA directory (Sweeny, 1978). Advertisers' indices in various clinical chemical and clinical pathology journals will also point to advertisements of manufacturers' kits. If the principle of the test or literature reference on which the test is based is not indicated there, the company or distributor should be contacted in order to select product(s) based on the methodology required. It would be advisable to obtain the literature usually packaged with the kits at this stage to narrow the field of choice.

Before making a final choice the literature should be checked to find whether any evaluations of these products have been published. Data from large-scale proficiency survey programs may also be helpful (see Section II, C, 1, c).

3. Kit Evaluation

The kit selection process is not really complete until it has been evaluated in the user's laboratory to determine whether it will successfully meet all the requirements that were set down for it at the outset. This is particularly necessary in order to assess if the performance or reliability characteristics can be met in the user's laboratory even though the manufacturer's data or other user's data might indicate that they should be met. There are four processes whereby this is done and they are (i) setting up specifications or performance standards for acceptable performance; (ii) performing evaluation experiments for precision, accuracy, specificity, and sensitivity; (iii) carrying out statistical analyses of the data; and (iv) finally judging the acceptability of the kit's performance.

A number of references have appeared in the literature outlining the experiments required to assess the performance of an analytical method (or kit) (Barnett, 1965; Barnett and Youden, 1970; Logan, 1972; Büttner *et al.*, 1979b; Broughton, 1978; Kim and Logan, 1978a; Lloyd, 1978; Neilsen and Ash, 1978; Westgard *et al.*, 1978b.) Rubin *et al.* 1979b; Vikelsöe et al. (1974).

a. Evaluation of Precision. As defined by the IFCC Committee on Standards (Büttner *et al.*, 1979a) *precision* is the agreement between replicate measurements and has no numerical value. Evaluation experiments are then designed to measure imprecision and expressed as the standard deviation or coefficient of variation. The first method developed for the evaluation of kit performance was that of Barnett (1965), which was subsequently revised (Barnett and Youden, 1970). Barnett's first evaluation of imprecision involved the analyses of purified analyte in solution at low, intermediate, and high levels relating to the usual levels of the constituents found in patients. These standard solutions were analyzed on each of 10 separate days by a reference method and by the kit procedure. In his revised procedure, Barnett carried out, in addition to aqueous standard analyses, day-to-day reproducibility studies on serum pools (usually commercial control sera of the same lot numbers) at three concentration levels over a period extended to 20 working days. He pointed out that estimates of day-to-day reproducibility are more meaningful than within-day or within-run reproducibility because in most clinical situations patients are tested only once a day or less often. Monitoring of the day-to-day reproducibility of the reference method is useful not only to compare the relative precision of the kit and reference methods but also to verify its adequacy since it is also used in the comparison method study for assessment of accuracy. Where it is necessary to limit the evaluation workload, the evaluation of imprecision of aqueous standards on a day-to-day basis may be omitted and the study carried out only on serum specimens.

Büttner *et al.* (1979b) recommended that factors, which contribute to imprecision, should be controlled as much as possible during the evaluation by using the same lot number of reagents, the same standards, instruments, and analysts. Stability of the specimens used for evaluation must be ensured over the evaluation period. This committee recommended the measurement of within-run imprecision by analyzing about 100 of patients' specimens in duplicate by the test method (kit) and by the comparison method making sure that the specimens chosen span the analytical ranges of both methods. The differences between duplicates are used to calculate the standard deviations for the two methods. The between-day imprecision is established by analyzing one sample of each of three control specimens (low, intermediate, and high values) placed in a random position in a run of patients' specimens, once per day for 20 consecutive working days. Stability over the test period must again be checked. The standard deviation of the 20 results is calculated.

Westgard *et al.* (1978b) also suggest that 20 test samples be used as the starting point for a replication experiment but if more data are needed, the experiment can be extended in time. They point out the possible interferences in some methods due to matrix effects with commercial control sera and thus compare within-run and within-day imprecision on both fresh patient samples and control specimens to see whether the matrix does have an effect. Their decision to monitor precision at analyte concentrations that are in the medically meaningful range, i.e., medical decision levels, is expedient. They state that it will generally be sufficient to identify the most critical medical situations and test two to four concentrations, which cover the analytical range of the method.

Neilsen and Ash (1978) recommend the documentation of both within-run and day-to-day imprecision at both a normal and elevated level. They suggest that the former study include not less than 30 replicate analyses on each of at least two concentrations and at least 40 replicate assays in the case of the latter, recording not more than two runs per day. Lloyd (1978) recommends three measures of imprecision: (i) *within-batch,* which measures the variability of the instrumentation and the operator; (ii) *between-batch,* which will reflect variations caused by variability of standards, instrument settings, etc., but not chemical variability between kits; (iii) *overall between-batch* to determine variability between batches of kits and reagents. Lloyd utilizes three specimens of material with concentrations of analyte at suitable levels and of sufficient quantity for at least 40 estimations. The specimens should preferably be of the fluid for which the kit is designed, and the concentrations should cover the analytical range of the kit and include clinically significant levels. Broughton (1978) points out that carryover of one sample to another is not confined to automated systems of analysis and is an important component of imprecision. He advises that replicates should be arranged in random positions in a run of patients' specimens, and not in a sequence, so that carryover effects are included. Kim and Logan (1978a) choose the day-to-day study as the best one to determine the degree of random error inherent in a particular kit in the hands of average laboratory operators. The importance of publishing details of the method for evaluating imprecision is stressed in their paper. They also advocate the use of more than one operator in kit evaluation to overcome any operator-induced bias and to more closely simulate conditions in a routine clinical chemistry laboratory. The authors recommend the checking of within-day imprecision at the initial, middle, and final stages of the evaluation period, using more than one laboratory operator. Care should be exercised in the choice of operators, i.e., only those with a proven record of good performance as judged by quality control results. The aim is to judge the performance of the kit without bringing into question the quality of the operator's skill in handling the product.

b. Evaluation of Accuracy. Barnett (1965) estimated accuracy of a kit in two ways: (i) performing recovery experiments and analyzing in triplicate analyte added at three different concentration levels to the base material and (ii) by analyzing 40 patients' specimens by both the kit and reference methods at a rate of not more than five tests per day. In the recovery experiments analyte levels were raised by approximately 20, 50, and 100% of normal levels. For the patient comparison study, Barnett and Youden (1970) recommend that for the 40 specimen values there should be a reasonably even distribution of the patient values into low, normal, and high ranges. They modified their original scheme in which outlier values beyond ± 3 SD were identified and eliminated to one in which these values were only eliminated when they were thought to be analytic errors on the basis of recalculation or recollection of improper procedure. Recovery experiments in the author's laboratory (Logan, 1972) were often carried out by weighing in analyte, where possible, to an ion-free serum as base material. Büttner et al. (1979b) recommend that simple tests for inaccuracy (e.g., linearity and recovery checks) should always be made before more complex procedures as undertaken. Since the accuracy

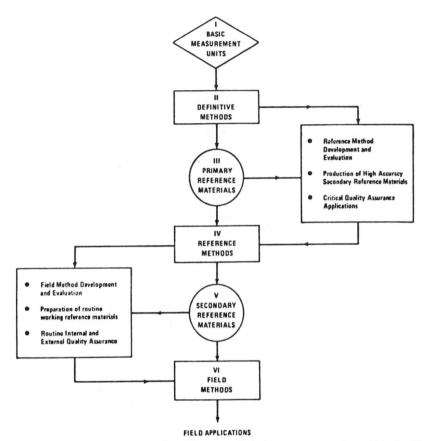

Fig. 1. Relationship among the different technical components of an "idealized" accuracy-based chemical measurement system.

of a set of results will be affected by errors of calibration, they prefer the use of the same set of calibration standards for both when two methods are compared. It is pointed out that recovery experiments will detect proportional bias, but not constant bias. They recommend that recovery experiments be made by adding varying amounts of pure material to each specimen and using as large a number of specimens as possible in order to include some containing potentially interfering substances. They also assess accuracy by comparing the values obtained by the test method (or kit) with those found with a comparison method of known accuracy. Patients' specimens (about 100) should be analyzed in replicate by both methods and these should be representative of those that a laboratory would expect to use with the kit. The selection of the comparison method is more important as it should be one that ideally would give true values for the assessment of accuracy.

The use of an accurate comparison method is a step in the accuracy transfer process, or what has now been developed as the systems approach to achieve compatible measurements among laboratories on a national (or international) scale. This approach is described in detail in the article by Uriano and Gravatt (1977), which reviews the role of reference materials and reference methods in chemical analysis. A schematic (Fig. 1) reproduced from their article illustrates the relationship among the different technical components of an "idealized" accuracy-based chemical measurement system. The basic measurement units are those seven base units described in the "Système International d'Unités" or SI System. In clinical chemistry, *definitive methods* are those which, after exhaustive investigation, are found to have no known source of inaccuracy (e.g., isotope dilution-mass spectrometry method for determining serum calcium). A *reference method* should have negligible bias or inaccuracy in comparison with the definitive method (e.g., the determination of serum calcium by atomic absorption spectroscopy, Cali *et al.*, 1973). *Field methods* refer to those methods of chemical analysis used in large volume applications on a routine basis. *Primary reference materials* are reference materials with properties certified by a recognized national standards laboratory (e.g., Standard Reference Materials, SRMs produced by the NBS). These are certified using definitive methods whenever possible. *Secondary reference materials* are those produced by commercial organizations or by individual laboratories for direct use as working standards. In many cases, these materials are directly related to SRMs or other primary reference materials. One example would be the secondary reference materials produced by CAP for use in laboratory survey programs. Büttner *et al.* (1979b) point out that reference methods in the true definition given above are only available in a few centers and may be laborious to use in fixing values to a wide range of patients' specimens. In Canada, the Canadian Society of Clinical Chemists has approved a number of "provisional reference methods" to serve in the interim until the "true" reference methods become available. In practice, it is more likely that values on control specimens certified by the reference method will be used for the accuracy transfer process.

Randell and Stevens (1977) recommend the use of three tests of accuracy: (i) assay before and after complete removal of the analyte; (ii) collecting all possible interfering substances (actual and potential) and processing these to establish the level of interference for each (a very impractical test); and (iii) comparison of results with those by a definitive or reference method on at least 50 samples of different levels of concentration.

Neilsen and Ash (1978) state that accuracy may be determined by comparison with a reference method, recovery experiments, and/or by analysis of reference materials. They express accuracy as a percentage figure using the absolute difference from the actual value. Accuracy should be determined over the usable concentration range of the assay using analytical grade reagents and NBS SRMs. Their recommendations for recovery experiments are similar to those of Barnett (1965), but they point out that 100% recovery does not necessarily indicate 100% accuracy. Lloyd (1978) describes two methods of assessing accuracy depending on whether or not the analyte being measured by the kit is available in a pure state. When the analyte is available in a pure form in sufficient quantities to be weighed, standard solutions in water or other suitable fluid may be prepared and these concentrations used as the true values. Five solutions covering the concentration range of the kit may be prepared and recoveries analyzed in triplicate. When it is not available in pure form, one must compare kit results with those obtained by a reference method. Where an internationally recognized reference method is not available, Lloyd suggests using a commonly used and understood technique for comparison. Broughton (1978) points out that the concept of accuracy is made more complex because of its relation to specificity (or dependence on the specimen) and the contributions made by different days, analysts, instruments, and laboratories. The latter factors may either be separated and regarded as components of inaccuracy or combined and become contributors to imprecision. He foresees the difficulty in developing definitive methods for complex molecules and in such cases arbitrary values may have to be assigned to standard materials by international agreement which, in turn, would be used to calibrate a well-defined method. Reference method values may be assigned to control specimens, which can then be used for testing accuracy of other methods. He finds that recovery experiments are difficult to interpret when results are approximately 95–105% and in such instances would recommend alternative procedures for assessing accuracy.

Kim and Logan (1978a) recommend the inclusion of patients' specimens in their 30-day precision study by analyzing two normal and two abnormal sera per day by the kit and reference methods. A total of 120 analyses is preferable using 30 grossly abnormal (hypo or hyper), 40 borderline, and 50 definitely normal. Westgard et al. (1978b) use the recovery experiment to estimate proportional analytical error. They use a test sample, which is prepared by adding a standard solution of the analyte to an aliquot of a patient sample. The baseline sample is prepared by adding solvent to a second aliquot of the sample so that the difference between the measured values of the two samples is the amount recovered. The volume of standard solution added must be kept small in comparison to the volume of the original patient sample in order that dilution of the matrix will not exceed 10%. These limitations would make it preferable to weigh in analyte where possible. Once again, these authors recommend the experiment be designed to assess recovery at the medical decision levels. Triplicate or quadruplicate analyses are generally necessary to obtain reliable results when the level of addition is small. More recovery experiments may be required when the comparison method used is not one of high quality. These authors state that the comparison of methods experiment to assess accuracy is often used to estimate systematic analytical error, without any regard to whether the error is constant or proportional. Reference methods are preferred for use in comparison experiments, but where this is not possible they recommend use of a method with known bias or systematic error and preferably one accepted professionally and in general use. At least 40 and preferably 100 patients' specimens should be analyzed in duplicate at a rate of two to five specimens per day. The specimens should be well chosen to represent the spectrum of diseases and cover the full range of analytical values expected in the routine use of the kit.

c. Evaluation of Specificity. Büttner *et al.* (1979a) define *specificity* as the ability of an analytical method to determine solely the component(s) it purports to measure and as such has no numerical value. Evaluation experiments are designed to measure interference that produce either low values for the analyte due to inhibition or high values due to enhancement. The magnitude of the effect depends on the concentration or amount of interfering material, but the relationship may not be proportional. The interference experiment can test if there are any effects from hemolysis, lipemia, or bilirubin, as well as specific substances known to cause particular problems for the determinations of interest.

Broughton (1978) differentiates between nonspecificity and interference. Nonspecificity causes inaccurately high results because the reaction cannot differentiate between the analyte and the interfering substance, e.g., a wide-band filter effect. In true interference the method is specific for the analyte, but inaccurate results are caused by an enhancement effect on the interfering material, e.g., depression of ionization of potassium by sodium ions in flame emission. Reagent and sample blanks can be used to control nonspecificity but are an unsatisfactory compromise. Neilsen and Ash (1978) urge that the influence of hemolysis, bilirubin, common laboratory anticoagulants, and capillary versus venous samples be documented at both normal and elevated concentrations. They suggest that aliquots of 30 patients' sera first be analyzed to determine baseline values and then be spiked with known amounts of the interfering substance and assayed in triplicate. Lloyd (1978) recommends the preparation of one solution of analyte in its source fluid containing no interfering substance and a second containing a high pathological concentration of it. Analyses are carried out in triplicate and if interference is found, solutions containing intermediate concentrations of the interfering substance are prepared and analyzed.

Westgard *et al.* (1978b) use the interference experiment to estimate systematic errors, constant in nature, arising when particular materials are added to the sample. A solution of material suspected to interfere is added to a solution of the analyte. A second solution is prepared by adding an equivalent amount of solvent to the analyte solution and analyzing both samples by the kit method. The authors point out that specificity can be tested separately by analyzing a solution of the interfering material without analyte. The suspected material should be added preferably near the maximum concentration expected in the patient population. The materials to be tested should be selected from literature reports and the listing by Young *et al.* (1975) is most useful for this purpose. They also recommend that interference samples also be analyzed by the comparative method, particularly when a routine service method has to be used in this capacity.

d. Evaluation of Sensitivity. The terms sensitivity and detection limit were defined by Büttner *et al.* (1979a). These same authors (1976b) point out that the term sensitivity commonly used to relate the ratio of the slope of the calibration curve to the standard deviation of replicate reading is a limited one resulting in ambiguous units. They describe the steps for determining detection limits using suitable blank samples known not to contain analyte. About 20 of these apparent blank samples are analyzed as well as a similar number of replicate samples with values near the blank-sample range. The limit calculated statistically at which a single result becomes significantly greater than the mean apparent blank-sample result is the detection limit (approximately equal to the mean $+2$ SD).

e. Statistical Approaches for Evaluation of Data. Several literature references (Barnett, 1965; Barnett and Youden, 1970; Barnett, 1971; Randell and Stevens, 1977; Kim and Logan, 1978b; Lloyd, 1978; Westgard *et al.*, 1974; Westgard, 1977; 1978c) are concerned with the statistical calculations to be used in processing the data obtained from evaluation of clinical chemistry methods (or kits). It will not be possible to consider in any detail the various statistical approaches that have been proposed, but it is hoped to trace the main advances that occurred since kit evaluations began. Barnett (1965) was the first to propose a scheme for the comparison of quantitative methods which included a protocol of the statistical manipulations to be applied to the evaluation data. The mean, standard deviation and range were calculated for the day-to-day precision results, mean percentage recoveries in the three spiked samples, the bias, standard deviation of the difference, and t values were calculated for the comparison experiment on 40 patient samples in the assessment of accuracy. Outliers beyond ± 3 SD in a plot of kit and reference method values were rejected from the data as large discrepancies. Groups of patients' specimens data were tested for runs and trends with time to locate any significant difference between groups. The revised scheme of Barnett and Youden (1970) includes modifications that permitted simplification of the statistical manipulations. The mean, standard deviation, and coefficient of variation were calculated for the day-to-day reproducibility based on 20 rather than 10 working days and included serum pools as well as aqueous standards. Barnett abandoned the statistical method for determining and eliminating outliers described in the original scheme, and discarded outliers only when recalculation or recollection of improper procedure indicated them to be analytic errors. In his revised procedure, the variance of the kit method was compared with that of the reference method for F test to determine statistical significance. The original serum pool value in the recovery experiments was calculated on the basis of 12 values instead of three as in the earlier paper. This application of statistics to patient comparison data, reproducibility studies, and recovery experiments is also contained in his textbook (Barnett, 1971).

Westgard and Hunt (1973) introduced the use of least-squares parameters as a statistical tool in treating the data from method comparison studies. This was a significant advance in that it allowed the evaluator to obtain specific estimates of proportional, constant, and random errors. By means of simulating different types of errors in test sets of data, these authors were also able to point out the limitations in using other statistical parameters such as bias, standard deviation of difference, and correlation coefficient. The t-test parameters of bias and standard deviation of difference provide estimates of constant and random errors, but only when proportional error is absent. The latter can only be estimated by means of least-squares analysis (i.e., calculation of slope of least-squares line, its y intercept, and the standard error of estimate along the y axis). The authors showed that comparison data must be presented graphically in order to detect limitations in least-squares analysis caused by nonlinearity and errant points. Westgard *et al.* (1978c) have continued since that time to develop a complete set of statistical calculations for all the aspects of evaluation of clinical chemistry methods (or kits). Their recent paper on statistics is one of a four-part series dealing with concepts and practices in the evaluation of clinical chemistry methods (Westgard *et al.*, 1978a,b,c,d). In this article, the authors discuss the application of the following statistical parameters to method evaluation: mean, standard deviation, coefficient of variation, standard error of the mean, paried *t* test, *F* test, linear regression analysis, and correlation coefficient. They point out that proper use and interpretation of statistics is essential if method (or kit) evaluation experiments are to provide objective decisions about the performance of a method. Their article first presents the equations used for calculating the above statistical parameters together with a discussion of their meaning. Second, the application of statistics to the comparison of methods experiment is discussed and compares the relative sensitivities of statistical parameters to different types of analytical error. In evaluation experiments aimed at estimating systematic errors, e.g., recovery and interference experiments, they recommend averaging results from several measurements or samples, since this will reduce the effects of random error inherent in the method. In discussing linear regression analysis, they consider one of its most useful applications to be the calculation of systematic error, which can be calculated for any concentration (e.g., a medical decision level) in the range of concentrations studied in the comparison of methods experiment. Their advice concerning outliers is to determine their cause rather than to eliminate them from the data by statistical means. If duplicate analyses are used for each method in the comparison study, the problem of outliers will be reduced.

Büttner *et al.* (1979b) recommend a sequence of steps to follow for comparison of methods statistically. The data pairs for the kit and comparison methods are plotted on a scatter diagram to check for linearity. The absolute differences of the pairs are then plotted against the mean of each pair and if these tend to increase with mean values, a logarithmic transformation of the data is carried out in order to equalize the variance. The linear regression line of Y (ordinate) on X (abscissa) is calculated statistically and the significance of the intercept value from zero is tested, i.e., whether the regression line passes through the origin. If it does pass through the origin, the logarithmic differences are used to calculate the mean and variation of the ratio Y/X. If the ratio differs more than negligibly from unity, a proportional bias exists. If the regression line does not pass through the origin, then the kit method is biased with respect to the comparison method. In the determination of detection limits, this committee recommends the calculation of the standard deviations of the blank samples and low samples, and then using a one-sided *t* test at $P = .01$ to calculate a detection limit which would be approximately equal to the mean blank result $+2.6$ SD

Randell and Stevens (1977) describe the statistical procedure for assessing the accuracy and precision of a method. They also plot the reference method values against the test method values and calculate the line of best fit or regression line. The intercept will be a measure of the sum of the systematic or constant errors whereas the slope will express how well the two methods correlate. They recommend the calculation of the correlation coefficient, r, which they state should have a value greater than $+0.98$ when comparing reference and definitive method results. For imprecision, they draw a histogram of the replicates (at least 30) to determine if the distribution is random. They test the goodness of fit of the data to that of an ideal distribution by means of Chi-square test. The smaller the figure for Chi-square the better is the fit. If the data do not fit, another function, i.e., log distribution, square root, etc., must be used to obtain a normal distribution before applying statistics. The mean and standard deviation are calculated when the normal distribution is obtained. The need to calculate SDs at different concentration levels is emphasized since these may vary with the concentration. The authors proceed to explain the use of the t test in comparing the results of two methods and in determining if their mean values differ significantly. They also outline the use of the F test to determine if there is any significant difference in the variance of the two methods. The authors fail to discuss the limitations of their statistical tools as was done by Westgard et al. (1978c).

Neilsen and Ash (1978) also stress that the SD and CV are meaningful measurements of imprecision only when there is a normal distribution of random analytical errors. They designate values outside ± 3 SD as outlier values and exclude them from the calculations. They state, however, that these should be specified along with the SD indicating what percent of the total values they represent. Lloyd (1978) eliminates from the statistical analysis any result falling at or beyond ± 4 SD from the mean as an outlier and reports it separately. He provides a list of 28 statistical equations together with definitions of the terms used in his scheme for evaluation of diagnostic kits. Lloyd recommends the presentation of results by different evaluators in a sufficiently standard way so that the performance of kits evaluated by different analysts may readily be compared. The mean, SD, and CV, are calculated to evaluate within-batch imprecision together with the 95% confidence limits for the mean and SD. The F test is recommended to determine if there is any significant difference in imprecision among reagent bottles within the batch. The SDs and confidence limits are also calculated when between-batch imprecision is being evaluated. A two-tailed t test is used to assess the significance of any apparent drift during the period of the evaluation. For linearity, graphs are plotted and linearity estimated taking into account the within-batch SD of the kit.

Lloyd also recommends the use of the least-squares regression line for the method comparison assessment of accuracy. He indicates that allowance for the imprecision of the reference method must be made in these accuracy comparisons. The slope of the regression line will indicate proportional error whereas the intercept will indicate any constant bias. When a kit method is being compared with a reference method, allowance must be made for the variance of the kit method to that of the reference method. Assuming this ratio is independent of the concentration of the analyte, estimates of the slope and intercept may be obtained from the statistical equations provided by Lloyd as well as the confidence limits for the slope. Confidence limits of the intercept cannot be determined in this situation.

Kim and Logan (1978b) present a new approach to the analysis of data obtained in the evaluation of methods (or kits) in clinical chemistry, which has application to kits generally but more especially to those designed to measure enzyme activity. In the calculation of day-to-day reproducibility they calculated the mean, SD, and CV from all data performed by two technologists and then removed data outside ±2 SD. The remaining screened data for each technologist were compared to determine if there was any significant difference in means or imprecision. The final mean, SD, and CV were determined for 20 screened data pooled from the first values in proportion to the total number of screened data each technologist performed. These edited data allowed imprecision comparison of each kit based on equal numbers of values and within 95% confidence limits of performance.

These authors designed a system of data analysis to overcome the problems of comparability of data generated from methods using different reaction conditions, units, and normal or reference values. Imprecision and comparative patient specimen data were converted to a normal range incorporated diagnostic index (DI) scale by the following equation:

Mean (test data), DIM

$$= \frac{test\ mean\ value - (\mathrm{MGNRH} + \mathrm{MGNRL}/2)}{\mathrm{MGNRH} - \mathrm{MGNRL}} \times 10$$

where DIM is the diagnostic index mean and MGNRH, MGNRL is the method given normal range, high and low limits, respectively.

This conversion to DI units results in the normal range mean ±2 SD for any constituent falling along a scale from −5 at the lower limit of the normal range to +5 at the upper limit. The establishment of a proper normal range is the key to success for this method of data treatment. In the comparison of methods, the above test (or kit) DI value is compared with the reference method DI value. This approach is designed to indicate if the kit problem is due to imprecision, lack of specificity, nonspecific inaccuracy, or an improperly established normal range. In order to determine if the problem is due to a poor selection of normal range by the kit manufacturer, the least-squares regression analysis is used to convert DI values to regressed data. These data are then substituted into the above equation replacing the method (or kit) given normal range (MGNRH and MGNRL) by that established for the reference method (RNRH and RNRL). The new diagnostic indices so obtained are called equalized diagnostic indices (EDI). The DI and EDI values are then compared with assessment criteria, PLD and PLV, described below (Section II, C, 3, f) to judge the acceptability of the kit method.

f. Performance Standards. Westgard (1977) has stated that the purpose of method evaluation is to judge whether the analytical performance of a laboratory method is acceptable. In order to do this, the amount of analytical error that is considered tolerable or allowable must be defined which, in turn, will depend on the clinical requirements of the test. Barnett (1968, 1971) and Tonks (1970) were perhaps among the first to try to set up what could be called performance standards with which to judge their evaluation and quality control data, respectively. Barnett developed tolerable coefficient of variation limits for 16 blood constituents, which he called medical significance values on the synthesis of opinions by clinicians and laboratory specialists. These values were applicable to 23 concentration levels (called decision levels) at which the clinician would be required to make a medical decision. Comparison of these coefficients of variation with those of the state of the art indicated those blood constituents for which more reliable methodology was required. Tonks proposed allowable limits of error (ALE) for a number of constituents commonly analyzed in the clinical chemistry laboratory. He divided a figure representing one-fourth of the normal range by the mean of the normal range and then multiplied this by 100 to convert the value to a percentage figure. The chief limitation of this figure was that it assumes that analytical error remains the same over the complete concentration range which, for most methods, is not the case. A more complete discussion of these performance standards has been given earlier (Logan, 1972).

Westgard *et al.* (1974) formulated criteria to judge if an analytical method (or kit) has acceptable precision and accuracy based on the medical usefulness of the test results. The analyst may think in terms of random and systematic error but the physician, on the other hand, thinks in terms of the total analytical error. This error, which is composed of both random and systematic errors, is medically more useful. Total error can then be used to formulate standards for acceptable performance. A

TABLE I

Performance Specifications Derived from Literature Sources

Test	Decision level (X_C) Barnett	Medically allowable error (E_A)				State-of-the-art limits		
		Barnett	Tonks	Gilbert	Cotlove	Duncan	Gilbert	Cresswell
Albumin	3.5 gm/dl	0.5			0.3	0.3		0.2
Bicarbonate	20 mmoles/liter	2.0			1.6			1.8
	30 mmoles/liter	2.0			1.6			1.8
Bilirubin	1.0 mg/dl	0.4						0.2
	20.0 mg/dl	3.0						
Calcium	11.0 mg/dl	0.5		0.55	0.32	0.60	0.79	0.36
Chloride	90 mmoles/liter	4.0	1.8	3.6	1.8	3.0	3.2	2.0
	110 mmoles/l	4.0	2.2	4.4	1.8		4.0	
Cholesterol	250 mg/dl	40	25	40	34	20	25	12.0
Creatinine	2.0 mg/dl			0.4		0.4	0.3	0.16
Glucose	50 mg/dl	10.0	5.0		9.0			6.0
	100 mg/dl	10.0	10.0	11.0	9.0		8.0	
	120 mg/dl	10.0	12.0	13.2	9.0		9.6	
Phosphate	4.5 mg/dl	0.5	0.45	0.5	0.46		0.39	0.24
Potassium	3.0 mmoles/liter	0.5		0.24	0.28	0.2	0.11	0.10
	6.0 mmoles/liter	0.5		0.48	0.28		0.23	
Sodium	130 mmoles/liter	4.0	2.3	3.8	1.0	3.0	3.1	2.0
	150 mmoles/liter	4.0	2.7	4.4	1.0		3.6	
Total protein	7.0 gm/dl	0.6	0.49	0.7	0.44	0.3	0.3	0.2
Urea nitrogen	27 mg/dl	4.0	2.7	5.0	3.0	6.0	4.2	2.4
Uric acid	6.0 mg/dl	1.0		0.9	1.1	0.4	0.36	0.28

specified value for total allowable error is interpreted as a 95% limit of allowable error (E_A). The medical decision level (X_C) is the concentration at which the performance of the method is critical. Westgard *et al.*, therefore, define performance standard (PS) as the allowable error (E_A) at the concentration (X_C) where critical medical decisions must be made. They point out that the evaluator, aided by performance standards derived from literature sources (Table I), must use professional judgment to decide on numerical values for E_A and X_c. The state-of-the art limits are valuable whenever medical usefulness requirements for a method are greater than the performance presently available. In this instance, more lenient values would need to be chosen so that not all methods would be judged unacceptable. The performance of a reference method might be helpful in such a case. A table of allowable CVs for the two medical situations in which an individual's test results are compared against those of a population group and against his own previous results has been prepared (Statland and Winkel, 1977), which could be used as guide for random error. No similar data for allowable inaccuracy are available.

Kim and Logan (1978b) have established two criteria to evaluate clinical chemistry methods for precision and accuracy. Permissible limits of variation (PLV) are used to assess precision whereas permissible limits of discrepancy (PLD) are used for assessing accuracy. These criteria have been developed empirically using both medically allowable errors and state-of-the art data available to the authors the sources of which are quoted in their paper. Two sets of PLV criteria were prepared, one for common clinical chemistry constituents and the other for special cases, e.g., electrolytes. Provision is allowed in these criteria for greater deviation on a sliding scale at EDI values for $+5$ for common constituents and above EDI values of -5 for the special group. In the case of the PLD criteria, the curves generated are most restrictive at the borderline values of DI $= +5$ and DI $= -5$. More generous limits on a sliding scale pertain at DI and EDI values higher and lower than these. Three curves are applied with both the PLV and PLD criteria and differentiate performance into four levels. The implication for both sets of criteria is that data generated by kits should not deviate beyond $\pm 25\%$ of the normal range span (i.e., ± 2.5 DI) from the target value.

g. Judging Acceptability of Performance. Once performance standards have been set that define the tolerable error for a method (or kit) at critical medical decision levels, the final procedure is to determine if the total analytical error found in the evaluation is greater than, equal to, or less than this amount. In earlier evaluations, judging acceptability of performance was very much a case of value judgment on the part of the laboratory director. Barnett (1971) compared the accuracy and precision of the kit method to that of the reference method and together with information on medical significance values (Barnett, 1968) reached a decision on the acceptability of the kit. Logan (1972) considered the number of false clinical decisions that would be generated by the kit values and considered these in a final judgment of acceptability. Not more than two were allowed in a series of 40 comparisons with a reference method.

Westgard and Hunt (1973), Westgard *et al.* (1974, 1978d) have provided the most complete set of criteria on which to judge the acceptability of the performance of a method (or kit). Performance is acceptable when the observed errors are smaller than the limit of allowable error (E_A) and not acceptable when they are greater. These authors formulate criteria based on clinical significance rather than statistical significance and are available for each type of analytic error. For random error (RE) obtained from the imprecision experiment, 1.96 SD of the kit method should be less than E_A for acceptability. For proportional error (PE), as estimated by the recovery experiment, the percentage error (% Recovery − 100) multiplied by the medical decision level, X_C, should be less than E_A. For constant error (CE) as obtained from the interference experiment, the bias of difference between results with and without addition of interfering material, should be less than E_A. Systematic error (SE) from the patient comparison study may be calculated at medical decision levels of interest X_C. By means of the regression line equation ($Y_C = A + BX_C$) the difference between the X and Y values ($Y_C - X_C$) or systematic error may be calculated. The total error (TE) is obtained by adding RE to SE and for a method (or kit) to be judged acceptable, this value should be less than E_A. If any of the above component errors exceed E_A, then the performance is unacceptable. Westgard describes two sets of performance criteria, one a single-value criteria, which may not be a reliable measure of the analytical error, and the second a better estimate called the confidence interval criteria which provides confidence intervals for the error estimates. Upper and lower 95% confidence limits, E_u and E_1, are generated. The E_u values are used to establish the criteria of acceptability whereas the E_1 values are used to establish the criteria for rejection, that is, $E_u < E_A$ and $E_1 > E_A$, respectively. When neither of these conclusions can be drawn, then more data are needed to provide a better estimate of analytical error. The authors point out that the application of these performance criteria to evaluation data depends on the assumption that the error distributions are gaussian in nature, that there is no error in the reference method, and that variance is uniform over the concentration range tested.

III. SPECIAL CONSIDERATIONS

A. Enzyme Kits

The evaluation of kits designed to measure enzyme activity in body fluids is more difficult than the evaluation of those that are produced to analyze the concentration of simple clinical chemistry constituents. Existing evaluation schemes can be applied to determine the precision of these kits, but the difficulty comes when trying to compare the performance of one kit against another or against a reference method. These difficulties are due to the wide variety of experimental conditions used among the methods and the units of measurement employed that are related to these methods. The calibrators most often used contain enzymes of animal origin that behave differently from the human ones present in the specimen being analyzed. Pure enzymes for recovery or accuracy studies are not available and in many cases reference methods for comparison experiments have not been developed.

Barnett (1972) proposed a method of treating data obtained from a patient comparison study in which alkaline phosphatase was measured kinetically by a reference procedure and also kinetically by a kit which employed entirely different units. The mean values for the two methods were calculated and a conversion factor obtained from the ratio of the reference mean to the kit mean. This factor was then used to equalize the vertical and horizontal scales and all the results were plotted so that each point represented the results by the two methods for each patient sample. Barnett *et al.* (1976) later applied this technique in a study of 43 GOT (AST) kits and was able to determine the correlations with the reference method in classifying the same patients as normal and abnormal. In his overall evaluation of these kits, Barnett scored the labeling, determined on about 60 patients' sera the number of false positives (test specificity), the number of false negatives (test sensitivity), day-to-day reproducibility over 20 days on normal and abnormal commercial control sera, and the relative standard deviation of the differences (S_d) between kit and reference results as a measure of accuracy on the patient sera. Acceptable performance was given for a labeling score of 14/19 or above, differences in test specificity and sensitivity not significantly different from the reference method by Chi-square test, CV $< 10\%$ and $< 7\%$ on the normal and abnormal pools, respectively, and relative $S_d < 15\%$. Only 5 out of the 43 kits met these criteria and were thus judged to be closely comparable to the reference method. Barnett also points out that disagreement in the numbers of false positives and false negatives from the reference method is an indication of normal values incorrectly assigned by the kit manufacturer. The scheme of Kim and Logan (1978b) makes it possible to identify kits with this shortcoming.

Grannis (1976, 1977) was faced with the task of developing an interlaboratory survey procedure for the CAP Chemistry Survey Program, which would allow meaningful performance evaluation of enzyme analyses. By spiking portions of a normal serum pool with creatinine, urea, and five enzymes and then preparing admixtures of the spiked pool with the original serum specimen, survey specimens bearing established linear interspecimen relationships as confirmed by creatinine and urea nitrogen analyses were prepared. Results were plotted as concentration units—in the case of creatinine and urea nitrogen and as enzyme activity units against the percentage of enzyme pool. The results were analyzed by linear regression to calculate the X intercept and slope to characterize the set of analyses. The individual laboratory results could either be compared with the appropriate mean X intercept and mean ratio of slopes for the applicable category or method constants could be derived to convert all results to comparative units. Two studies of this kind in 10 and 40 laboratories have been sufficiently promising to initiate a survey open to several hundred laboratories. Thus a method whereby the performance of enzyme kits, in particular their accuracy, may be evaluated with a high degree of confidence seems imminent.

Westgard *et al.* (1975) describe an evaluation protocol that is designed specifically for testing methods, which measure enzyme activity using aspartate aminotransferase (AST) methods as an example. The authors first of all defined the application, methodology, and performance characteristics which must be considered in assessing the suitability of the AST methods. Definitions of these were given in Sections II, C, 1a,b, and c. Under performance characteristics they list as the most essential for inclusion in the testing protocol, precision, assay range, substrate depletion check, freedom from interferences, and accuracy as tested by comparison with a reference method. Temperature control, timing, reagent, and product stability could be tested, but their effects are reflected by precision and accuracy studies. The authors pass final judgment on the acceptability of the enzyme method (or kit) performance by comparing the total analytic error with the allowable error (E_A) at a medical decision level (X_C) recommended for enzyme activity measurement to be slightly above the upper limit of the expected range for normals (Westgard *et al.*, 1978d). Their evaluation protocol requires testing of within-run precision (20 replicates), linearity, substrate depletion error using a high activity specimen, interferences trying materials listed by Young *et al.* (1975), between-run and total between-day precision, and accuracy by comparison of 48 patient specimen results with those of a reference method. The protocol allows for the simultaneous testing of up to 4 kits over an 8-week period. The statistical analysis procedure is similar to that employed for other clinical chemistry methods (Westgard *et al.*, 1978c).

Broughton (1978) states that selection of a reliable method for enzyme assay is difficult due to the many interrelated variables that must be considered. They all affect enzyme activity and results are always entirely method dependent. Continuous monitoring methods are preferable because they allow the selection of the initial linear portion of the reaction curve and enable the progress of the reaction to be followed. An enzyme standard must behave in exactly the same way as the enzyme in human serum with the same optima and temperature effects, and minor changes in assay procedure must produce the same effect on results. Where the standard is of human origin, Broughton notes that difficulties can arise in selecting the isoenzyme to use. He concludes that a universal calibration material for an enzyme may not be possible, but further information about their commutability effects would enable methods to be selected in which these differences had the least influence on results. International activity has been directed toward standardization, particularly of temperature, for enzyme assays (Bowers and McComb, 1975).

As mentioned in Section II, C, 3, f Kim and Logan (1978b) devised a scheme of converting enzyme activity measurements to diagnostic (DI) and equalized diagnostic units in order to compare the results of kits with each other and a reference method. This scheme was applied by Pryce *et al.* (1977) to an evaluation study of 19 kits designed to measure creatine phosphokinase (CPK) activity. One of the chief advantages of the DI conversion is that it allows the evaluator to assess the suitability of the normal range assigned by the manufacturer to the kit. The development of PLV and PLD criteria (Section II, C, 3, f), for definitions) provides limits for imprecision and inaccuracy for assays of enzyme activity that show flexibility with increasing activity. In the case of PLD, these provide the evaluator with some guidance in determining the acceptability or rejection of systematic error.

B. Radioimmunoassay Kits

As mentioned above (Section I, A), the increase in RIA kits on the market in the last 5 years has been phenomenal. As these kits are based on a competitive protein-binding principle of assay incorporating the use of radioisotope material, special consideration should be given to criteria for their selection.

Griffiths and Logan (1974) discussed the commercial availability, standardization, and quality control of clinical diagnostic RIA tests and reagents. They pointed out the problems encountered in standardization, particularly for human protein hormones due to the complex structure of the proteins. Limited immunological cross-reactivity of these human hormones with similar hormones from other species requires that standardization be carried out with materials obtained from human sources. Most glycoproteins contain more than one immunoreactive group, which creates a specificity problem. Evidence that a particular organ-derived hormone has a different chemical composition from the similar hormone originating from other parts of the body is another complication. Problems such as these place serious restrictions on the collection of appropriate substances for reference standards and antigens for antiserum production. The hormones TSH, FSH, LH, and CG contain α- and β-subunits jointed in noncovalent linkage. The similar chemical structures of the α subunits in these hormones probably accounts for the high incidence of immunological cross-reactivity among them. These authors pointed out the need for reference RIA methods using standardized hormone preparations and antisera in order to properly assess the accuracy of RIA kits by the comparative method technique as applied in the more common chemistry constituent assays (Section II, C, 3 b). They discussed the quality control of RIA measurements and recommended the parameters suggested by Rodbard *et al.* (1968) be examined. Examination of these same parameters may be applied to evaluating the performance of a RIA kit.

Walker (1977) published an excellent review article designed to assist analysts with limited experience in immunoassay. He points out that immunoassay has more experimental variables than most other analytical techniques and sets out to show which variables have most effect on the outcome of the test. Imprecision is emphasized, seldom better than $\pm 5\%$ CV for within-batch and $\pm 10-15\%$ for between-batch. There are many practical details discussed in relation to radioimmunoassays which would be useful in kit selection. As an example, he recommends use of solid-phase antibody separation for small numbers of samples and charcoal or second antibody for larger batches. The former would be used for steroids whereas the latter would be used for digoxin and polypeptides.

Spierto and Shaw (1977) describe the problems that affect RIA procedures and this information can be particularly useful in the selection of a RIA kit. They found from interlaboratory and intralaboratory studies that the imprecision for laboratories using RIA procedures was much higher than that for laboratories using conventional procedures. The most critical step in RIA procedures is the separation of the antibody-bound antigen from the free antigen. This is a physical separation using an adsorbent such as dextran- or protein-coated charcoal to remove the free fraction. This action upsets the original equilibrium between the bound and free fractions and can be a major source of error unless the separation can be effected quickly and reproducibly. The authors reported on a number of experiments with charcoal-separating agents and found that both the amount of charcoal and coating agent must be carefully chosen. Proteins present in the unknown samples can coat the charcoal so that variable levels of serum proteins in the samples can introduce a significant error. They also reported that the method of radioiodination of antigen can result in a product in which not all the label is associated with immunoreactive antigen but with free iodide or deteriorated nonreactive antigen, which increases with storage time. Specificity of the antibody for the antigen to be measured is most important and RIA procedures can suffer from specific interferences due to hormonal cross-reactivity and nonspecific factors. The latter are hard to control since they may be present in patients' sera but not in the solutions used to prepare calibration curves. The reduction of RIA data can also introduce a source of error. Since the percentage of radioactivity bound to antibody when plotted against the concentration of unlabeled antigen is nonlinear, a logit transformation as proposed by Rodbard (1974) is often used to linearize the data. It may introduce error especially at the extremes of the dose–response curve.

Witherspoon (1976) has produced a protocol for the evaluation of commercial RIA kits. At the same time he has provided much useful information about sources of error and differences one may find in kits and on how to select one suitable for the laboratory from the large number now commercially available. Labeled standards and binding characteristics of antisera may differ from kit to kit. Procedural differences such as equilibrium or nonequilibrium incubation, separation techniques, and temperature dependence may significantly alter the results. For example, the author indicates that as many as nine different separation techniques are offered among 30 different commercial thyroxine kits. He recommends the following steps in the choice of a kit:

1. Understand well the physiology and pathophysiology of the analyte and its concentration fluctuations in the biological material of interest so that test requirements may be well formulated.
2. Check literature that may provide any information on the advantages of one method over another.
3. Obtain procedure protocols and package inserts from kit manufacturers to determine the method principle, the material supplied, what the user has to provide by way of other materials and equipment.
4. The manufacturer's literature should identify the standard material

and state its equivalence to recognized international standards, if available.

5. All kit components should be clearly identified with lab numbers, contents, and when applicable, concentrations, amounts of radioactivity, and specific activities.

6. Storage conditions and expiration dates should be clearly stated.

7. The precautions for handling, and if possible, the personnel hazards should be clearly stated.

8. Validation data should be provided, including assessment of method sensitivity, imprecision, inaccuracy, and specificity. The WHO Expert Committee on Biological Standardization (1975) has suggested that this include, where possible, data as follows: representative dose–response curve, and summary statistics for such curves from several repetitive assays, antibody dilution curve, cross-reactivity data, parallelism of standard and unknown recovery experiments, within-and between-assay imprecision, Scatchard plots and equilibrium constants, time–temperature data, comparison with other methods of assay, detailed information on all parameters likely to affect assay performance, physiological or clinical data to substantiate intended use, literature references, and range of normal and pathological values.

9. Request a trial kit for initial evaluation of the one most likely to be suitable.

Witherspoon also provides an evaluation protocol to validate the data supplied by the manufacturer and which should be completed before accepting the kit for routine use. Inaccuracy is assessed in three ways by generating and comparing standard dose curves with the kit standard and reference standard material, by determining recovery of known standard added to human serum at three dose levels, and by performing a comparative study with a reference or previous reliable method. Within-run imprecision is obtained by making 10 replicate measurements on high and low control samples within the same assay. Later between-run imprecision can be estimated on control specimens assayed in different runs. Within-run CV for RIA procedures may be 5–10% and between-run CV as high as 10–20%. To determine sensitivity, 10 replicates of the maximum binding sample, i.e., no added unlabeled ligand are assayed and the minimum detection limit is calculated. The shape and slope of the standard curve are examined to find the point of maximum sensitivity on the standard dose–response curve. To check specificity a high patient sample is diluted and plotted to verify parallelism of a dose–response curve for dilutions with the standard curve. Cross-reactivity can be evaluated by measuring patients' samples thought to cross-react with the material which the assay is designed to measure. Finally, patient samples of known high and low concentrations of analyte are assayed to evaluate the correctness of the normal range provided by the manufacturer. It is always necessary for the user to establish values for the local patient population whether or not they agree with values supplied by the manufacturer.

IV. RECOMMENDED CRITERIA FOR KIT SELECTION

A. Process of Kit Selection

The process of selection of a kit for use in the clinical chemistry laboratory is only one part of the larger task of selecting the most suitable analytical method. In this case, part of the selection process has been completed with the decision for whatever reason that the laboratory test should be undertaken using commercially produced diagnostic reagents along with the manufacturer's test procedure. Even though the selection process may have proceeded this far, all criteria used in the larger process are still very applicable and will be contained in the recommendations. The process of method (or kit) selection consists in (1) defining the requirements for the method; (2) determining from the literature what methods are available; and (3) choosing the method that has the best chance of meeting the defined requirements. The decision to use a kit rather than a classical manual procedure from the literature would be reached during this three-step process of method selection. The three steps, however, may well be repeated in determining, from among the products available on the market, the kit most likely to fulfill the laboratory's requirements. The selection process to this point has to be made entirely on what information the analyst has been able to assemble regarding the characteristics of the kit. This is accomplished by reading the various manufacturers' kit inserts, evaluation reports in the literature, and listening to experiences related by colleagues. This leads to the choice of a kit for trial in the laboratory, but the selection process cannot really be considered complete until the kit's performance has been evaluated in the analyst's laboratory and found to be acceptable. If the first kit is unacceptable then a second selection must be made and the laboratory evaluation repeated.

The first and essential step before any selection of a method (or kit) can be made is to carefully define what is required of the method. In other words, what characteristics must it have if it is to achieve its purpose in the laboratory. These characteristics are of two classes: (1) practicability characteristics such as types of specimens, speed, technical skill requirements, operational requirements, service requirements, safety, cost, etc. and (2) reliability characteristics such as chemical specificity, chemical sensitivity, precision, and accuracy. Westgard *et al.* (1978a) calls the first application characteristics and divides the second equally into methodology and performance characteristics thus creating three classes instead of two. All of the required characteristics may not be found in any one product available. The analyst then must select the one that has best balance for the laboratory in which it is to be used. A careful choice as to which characteristics are most important must, therefore, be made. The criteria for kit selection in relation to practicability and reliability characteristics will be considered separately.

B. Criteria Related to Practicability

The practicability characteristics are factors of primary importance in determining if it is practical to utilize the kit in the particular laboratory under consideration. The definition of the method requirements as they relate in turn to these characteristics provides the necessary information by which a judgment may be made concerning the suitability of the kit (i.e., criteria for selection). The establishment of the requirements for the kit as related to these characteristics are listed below. In such cases the criterion for selection is the answer to the question, "Does this product meet the requirement for the test as defined for our laboratory?"

1. *Specimen.* Determine the types of patients for whom the measurement will be requested, the type of specimen, i.e., serum, plasma, spinal fluid, urine, etc., and the volumes of samples available. Select those kits meeting these requirements.
2. *Speed.* Establish the rate at which specimens should normally be processed for analyses of this constituent in the laboratory. Establish the tolerable time intervals between presentation of the specimen to the analyst and the availability of the result in the two cases when the analyst is and is not prepared for it. If speed of analyses can be varied for the test, find out what effect this may have on accuracy and precision. This information may not be available for the kit and may have to be assessed in the laboratory.
3. *Technical skill.* Compare the complexity of the kit techniques available for the test to determine the levels of technical skill required. Determine how much training may be needed to learn each technique. Selection should be made on the basis of simplicity where

possible as the more complex the procedure the greater likelihood of analytical error.

4. *Operational.* Examine the manufacturers' inserts provided with the kits to assess if the detail and clarity of instructions are sufficient to avoid different analysts interpreting them in different ways thus introducing their own modifications and making assessments valueless. Determine if the kit has any operational requirements that preclude its use in the laboratory. Establish if any instrumentation is required to be provided for the kit technique that is not available in the laboratory. Where additional equipment is required to perform the kit test, it should be readily available, e.g., need for special sample containers. Determine if all reagents are provided in the kit by the manufacturer and if not, whether they are readily available. Select kits using reagents of good quality and stability. Examine their formulation to ascertain if reagents present any problems in handling, waste disposal, pollution, etc. The frequency of reordering reagents on the basis of kit test capacity should be determined. Select the kit with the most favourable operational requirements particularly where technical skill may be limited.

5. *Service.* Service requirements would probably only be a consideration for those kits designed to be used with a special instrument system. In these cases, one would need to know if there were any special requirements for power supply, ventilation, temperature, or humidity control, etc. The selection should be for a kit and analyzer system compatible with the services already available in the laboratory area. A system also with the best record as to mechanical breakdown and need for expert technical servicing should be selected. This characteristic has also been called dependability.

6. *Safety.* A kit should be selected that presents the least hazard to the operator or other staff in the area. Where it is necessary to use a kit that presents a hazard, the manufacturer's instructions should give adequate warning of this and the action to be taken in the case of a spill or other instance of maximum exposure. Select kits which present the least hazard due to toxicity, radioactivity, flammability, explosion, carcinogenicity, or generation of infectious aerosols.

7. *Cost.* Select a kit for which the cost per actual test specimen is reasonable based on its reagent constitution. Experience has shown that the prices charged may vary greatly among products with no apparent relation to the cost of chemicals required to make up the kit. When the cost per test is calculated, including technologist time, comparisons should be made for cost at the maximum rate at which specimens can be processed, for smaller workloads and for a single

specimen. Selection will have to be made in relation to what is considered a tolerable cost per test in the analyst's laboratory.

C. Criteria Related to Reliability

The reliability characteristics are those factors of the method (or kit) that describe the chemical properties on which the procedure is based and which demonstrate how reliably the method performs. In order to apply criteria for kit selection related to these characteristics, one must again define the laboratory's requirements for these parameters at the outset.

1. *Choice of chemical reaction.* This is probably one of the very first decisions that the analyst makes at the beginning of the selection process. His choice will be a method based on the chemical principle that is most likely to provide the chemical specificity and sensitivity and the analytical performance required for the particular analyte. It is following this choice that he can determine if commercial kits are indeed available that are based on this chemical reaction. It will usually be necessary to obtain manufacturers' literature inserts to establish the chemical principle and the literature references on which the kit method is based. Select those kits utilizing that principle and look further in the technical literature for any evaluation reports or ask the kit distributor for names of any users so that they may be consulted.

2. *Assay conditions.* The temperature at which the assay is performed is another consideration in the selection of a kit. Assays conducted at 25°C may not be satisfactory in some laboratories due to the difficulty in maintaining this temperature. It will be necessary to select a kit whose assay conditions can be most readily provided in the laboratory. It should also be determined that under these conditions the reaction of the kit method is linear with respect to the concentration of analyte.

3. *Calibration.* The manner of calibration of the kit procedure is important and should be examined to see if it is scientifically valid to ensure accuracy. Avoid using kits having serum standards as their specificity may be suspect and they are difficult to calibrate accurately. Laboratory verification of the standard provided against a NBS SRM is the only sure way.

4. *Analytical range.* The analytical range required for the method can be established on the basis of ranges of concentrations expected in the patient population. Only those kits that provide evidence of linearity over the required range in the manufacturers' inserts should be selected.

5. *Precision*. The precision of the method is established on the basis of what is required to provide clinically useful results and in particular at the medical decision levels. Check the data provided in the inserts and in particular that shown for between-day imprecision. Check the adequacy of the data on which the calculations have been made. Choose a kit with a documented performance indicating a level of imprecision less than or at least equivalent to that needed for the test. This is one of the parameters that will have to be experimentally verified.

6. *Recovery*. The experimental data provided on recovery enables the analyst to determine if a proportional bias exists in the kit procedure. The data obtained from the manufacturer should be examined and only those kits with bias less than or equal to that tolerable for the analytical procedure should be selected. Constant bias is not measured in recovery experiments.

7. *Interference*. The manufacturer should document at least the effect of common interfering materials on the kit procedure and the data should be examined to see if they are sufficient to validate the statements made about interference. Kits selected should be those subject to the least interference by these materials keeping in mind the nature of the specimens expected from the patient population. Where interference does exist, the decision must be taken as to whether it is tolerable or a correction can be made which will not invalidate the results.

8. *Specificity*. The manufacturers' inserts should be examined for information on the limitations of specificity in the kit procedure. The system of blanking should provide corrections for nonspecificity, i.e., a reagent blank to correct for the contribution of the reagents to sample readings and a sample blank to compensate for the reading given by substances other than the analyte. Kit methods that are the most specific should be selected and where problems due to nonspecificity exist these should be adequately described and proper blanking procedures provided in the manufacturers' protocols.

9. *Accuracy*. Accuracy is the agreement between the best estimate of a quantity and its true value. The measurement of inaccuracy by comparing values obtained by the kit procedure with those by a reference method is the systematic error and the data provided in the manufacturers' inserts should be examined to see if they are adequate and whether the bias obtained is tolerable for the given laboratory requirement.

10. *Detection limit*. The kit procedure should indicate the detection

limit or smallest single result that can be distinguished statistically from a blank. Only those kits possessing sufficient sensitivity to detect adequately the smallest concentration of the constituent that would be of medical significance should be selected.

11. *Robustness.* Some indication of the robustness of the kit procedure may be gained if the manufacturer has provided information on collaborative testing or if there is information in the literature (e.g., evidence of acceptable performance in most laboratories in large proficiency testing surveys) that it can withstand transfer from one laboratory to another without alteration in the quality of the results obtained with it.

D. Laboratory Evaluation for Kit Selection

To make the final selection of a kit, the analyst requires complete information on the practicability and reliability characteristics of the kit in order to assess its quality. If adequate information is not provided by the manufacturer or is unavailable in the literature, the analyst must evaluate it in his laboratory in order to provide the quantitative data for an objective judgment. Even if it is readily at hand, the variability of laboratory environments and of technical skills available makes it highly desirable for the analyst to confirm these findings in his laboratory. The criteria to be applied are the same as discussed above, i.e., to determine if the performance of the kit is acceptable with respect to the laboratory's needs for the particular type of analysis.

It is not the intention to describe herein the step-by-step experimental and statistical procedures to be applied in the kit evaluation process as these are described elsewhere, perhaps most fully, by Westgard (1978a,b,c,d) and will be covered in IFCC recommendations for commonly determined chemical chemistry constituents as glucose, urea, total bilirubin, total protein, albumin, and hemoglobin (Logan et al. 1981b). For special evaluation procedures such as enzymes and RIA tests, the reader is referred to the work of Barnett (1976), Kim and Logan (1978), Westgard *et al.* (1975), and Witherspoon (1976).

A valid assessment can only be made by staff with appropriate training and relevant experience. The general approach to kit evaluation uses similar principles to those recommended for the evaluation of analytical methods for routine use (Büttner *et al.*, (1979b). The various stages may be summarized as follows:

1. Assess the product labeling and accompanying literature using a 20-point score sheet developed from the WHO labeling recommendations (Logan *et al.*, 1981a).

2. Prepare calibration solutions, assemble the equipment required, and test out the kit method in a preliminary manner until familiarity with the test is gained (Logan *et al.*, 1981b).
3. Assess linearity, analytical range, within-run, and within-day imprecision. Check on recovery and estimate proportional error. Assess possible interferences (Logan *et al.*, 1981b). The initial performance of the kit may be assessed at this stage to determine if a full evaluation should be carried out (Westgard *et al.*, 1978c,d).
4. The following may be done concurrently: (a) assess between-day imprecision over 20 working days (Logan *et al.*, 1981b). (b) Set up a comparison method and assess the relative inaccuracy of the kit method by analyzing 50–100 patient specimens by both methods over 20 working days. Calculate constant error, proportional error, and total error (Westgard *et al.*, 1978b).
5. Evaluate the overall performance of the kit using the performance standards set in the laboratory for the particular test and using the criteria of acceptable performance developed by Westgard *et al.* (1978d).

It is recommended that tests should be done in the above order so that the evaluation may be terminated and the kit rejected at any stage if the results obtained are considered unsatisfactory. Thus, final selection must await the evaluation of performance in the user's laboratory since the first commercial kit tested may not meet the requirement defined at the outset.

V. CONCLUSIONS

The analyst must continue to make decisions on the suitability of commercial kits for the clinical chemistry laboratory in view of the diversity and multitude of such products available on the market. Although regulatory controls in North America have been responsible for improvement among the products offered, their emphasis on verification of manufacturers' claims does not always ensure the user that the kit will perform satisfactorily to the clinical requirements of a given laboratory or institution. Criteria for kit selection that have been published are reviewed, i.e., the labeling and enclosed literature, the practicability, and reliability characteristics. The special considerations that have been published for the assessment of enzyme and radioimmunoassay kits are also reviewed.

Although certain criteria may be applied to the manufacturers' brochures and inserts and to the published literature in making preliminary selections a final choice cannot be made without the user defining the requirements of the given laboratory situation and carrying out a product evaluation in the laboratory. Criteria recommended for kit selection have been developed that take into consideration all these aspects of the selection process.

REFERENCES

AACC Committee on Standards and Controls (1966). *Clin. Chem. (N.Y.)* **12**, 43–44.

Barnett, R. N. (1965). *Am. J. Clin. Pathol.* **43**, 562–569.

Barnett, R. N. (1968). *Am. J. Clin. Pathol.* **50**, 671–676.

Barnett, R. N. (1971). "Clinical Laboratory Statistics." Little, Brown, Boston, Massachusetts.

Barnett, R. N. (1972). *Prog. Clin. Pathol.* **4**, 181–198.

Barnett, R. N. (1977). *In* "Laboratory Medicine" (G. J. Race, ed.), Vol. I, Chapter 20. Harper and Row, Hagerstown, Maryland.

Barnett, R. N., and Youden, W. J. (1970). *Am. J. Clin. Pathol.* **54**, 454–462.

Barnett, R. N., Ewing, N. S., and Skodon, S. B. (1976). *Clin. Biochem.* **9**, 78–84.

Bostick, W. D., and Mrochek, J. E. (1977). *Clin. Chem. (N.Y.)* **23**, 1633–1639.

Bowers, G. N., and McComb, R. B. (1975). *Clin. Chem. (N.Y.)* **21**, 1988–1995.

Broughton, P. M. G. (1978). *Prog. Clin. Pathol.* **7**, 1–31.

Brown, D. J. (1976). *Am. J. Clin. Pathol. Suppl.* **66**, 223–233.

Büttner, J., Borth, R., Boutwell, J. H., Broughton, P. M. G. and Bowyer, R. C. (1979a). Clin. Chim. Acta 98, 129F–143F.

Büttner, J., Borth, R., Boutwell, J. H., Broughton, P. M. G. and Bowyer, R. C. (1979b). Clin. Chim. Acta. 98, 145F–162F.

Cali, J. P., Bowers, G. N., and Young, D. S. (1973). *Clin. Chem. (N.Y.)* **19**, 1208–1213.

Carey, R. N., Feldbruegge, D., and Westgard, J. O. (1974). *Clin. Chem. (N.Y.)* **20**, 595–602.

Chong-Kit, R., and McLaughlin, P. (1974). *Clin. Chem. (N.Y.)* **20**, 1454–1457.

Chua, K. S., and Tan, I. K. (1976). *J. Clin. Pathol.* **29**, 517–519.

Crowley, L. V., and Alton, M. (1971). *Am. J. Clin. Pathol.* **56**, 636–644.

Edwards, C. C. (1973). *Fed. Regist.* **38**, 7096–7102.

Fingerhut, B. (1978). *Clin. Chem. (N.Y.)* **24**, 1624–1627.

Galen, R. S., and Gambino, S. R. (1975). "Beyond Normality: The Predictive Value and Efficiency of Medical Diagnosis." Wiley, New York.

Grannis, G. F. (1976). *Am. J. Clin. Pathol. Suppl.* **66**, 206–222.

Grannis, G. F. (1977). *Am. J. Clin. Pathol. Suppl.* **68**, 142–152.

Griffiths, B. W., and Logan, J. E. (1974). Health Protection Branch/Industry Research Seminar, Ottawa.

Haeckel, R. (1976). *J. Clin. Chem. Clin. Biochem.* **14**, 227–237.

Henry, P., and Saunders, R. A. (1975). *Ann. Clin. Biochem.* **12**, 119–125.

IJpma, S. T., Blijenberg, B. G., and Leijnse, B. (1978). *Clin. Chem. (N.Y.)* **24**, 489–492.

Kim, E. K., and Logan, J. E. (1978a). *Clin. Biochem.* **11**, 238–243.

Kim, E. K., and Logan, J. E. (1978b). *Clin. Biochem.* **11**, 244–250.

Krynski, I. A., and Logan, J. E. (1968). *Clin. Biochem.* **2**, 105–114.

Lam, C. W. K., and Tan, I. K. (1978). *Clin. Chem. (N.Y.)* **24**, 143–145.

Lloyd, P. H. (1978). *Ann. Clin. Biochem.* **15**, 136–145.

Loeb, W. F., and Bauman, G. (1971). *J. Am. Vet. Med. Assoc.* **159**, 1108–1111.

Logan, J. E. (1972). *CRC Crit. Rev. Clin. Lab. Sci.* **3**, 271–289.

Logan, J. E., and Sunderland, M. L. E. (1970). *Clin. Chem. (N.Y.)* **16**, 990–997.

Logan, J. E., and Taada, D. R. (1977). *Clin. Biochem.* **10**, 133–137.

Medical Devices Regulations, Food and Drugs Act. (1975). *Can. Gazette,* Part II, *No.* 18, **109**, 2491–2498.

National Committee for Clinical Laboratory Standards (1975). "Approved Standard: ASL-1." NCCLS, Villanova, Pa.

National Committee for Clinical Laboratory Standards (1980). "Tentative Standard: TSLA;1." NCCLS, Villanova, Pa.

Neilsen, L. G., and Ash, K. O. (1978). *Am. J. Med. Technol.* **44**, 30–37.

Passey, R., Gillum, R. L., Giles, M. L., and Fuller, J. B. (1975). *Clin. Chem. (N.Y.)* **21**, 1108–1112.

Pearson, J. R. (1978). *Clin. Chem. (N.Y.)* **24**, 1823–1825.

Porter, W. H., and Roberts, R. E. (1978). *Clin. Chem. (N.Y.)* **24**, 1620–1624.

Pryce, F. H., Kim, E. K., and Logan, J. E. (1977). *Clin. Biochem.* **10**, 206–209.

Randell, J. A., and Stevens, J. F. (1977). Institute of Medical Laboratory Sciences Current Topics in Medical Laboratory Sciences, No. 1, 1–12.

Rodbard, D. (1974). *Clin. Chem. (N.Y.)* **20**, 1255–1270.

Rodbard, D., Rayford, P. L., Cooper, J. H., and Ross, G. T. (1968). *J. Clin. Endocrinol. Metab.* **28**, 1412–1418.

Rubin, M., Barnett, R. N., Bayse, D., Beutler, E., Brown, S. S., Logan, J., Reimer, C., Westgard, J. O., and Wilding P. (1979a). *Clin. Chim. Acta,* **95**, 155F–162F.

Rubin, M., Barnett, R. N., Bayse, D., Beutler, E., Brown, S. S., Logan, J., Reimer, C., Westgard, J. O., and Wilding, P. (1979b). *Clin. Chim. Acta,* **95**, 163F–168F.

Spierto, F. W., and Shaw, W. (1977). *CRC Crit. Rev. Clin. Lab. Sci.* **8**, 365–372.

Statland, H. E., and Winkel, P. (1977). *In* "CAP Aspen Conference 1976: Analytical Goals in Clinical Chemistry" (F. R. Elevitch, ed.) pp. 94–101. College of American Pathologists, Skokie, Illinois.

Sunderland, M. L. E., and Logan, J. E. (1971). *Clin. Biochem.* **4**, 22–28.

Sunderland, M. L. E., Kim, E. K., and Logan, J. E. (1972). *Clin. Biochem.* **5**, 186–193.

Sweeny, M. (1978). *Lab. World No. 8* **29**, 48–70, 84–89.

Tonks, D. B. (1970). "Quality Control in Clinical Laboratories," Diagnostic Reagents Division, Warner-Chilcott Laboratories Co. Limited, Scarborough, Ontario.

Uriano, G. A., and Gravatt, C. C. (1977). *CRC Crit. Rev. Anal. Chem.* **6**, 361–410.

Vikelsöe, J., Bechgaard, E., and Magid, E. (1974). *Scand. J. Clin. Lab. Invest.* **34**, 149–152.

Walker, W. H. C. (1977). *Clin. Chem. (N.Y.)* **23**, 384–402.

Westgard, J. O. (1977). *In* "CAP Aspen Conference 1976: Analytical Goals in Clinical Chemistry" (F. R. Elevitch, ed.), pp. 105–114. College of American Pathologists, Skokie, Illinois.

Westgard, J. O., and Hunt, M. R. (1973). *Clin. Chem. (N.Y.)* **19**, 49–57.

Westgard, J. O., Carey, R. N., and Wold, S. (1974). *Clin. Chem. (N.Y.)* **20**, 825–833.

Westgard, J. O., Carey, R. N., Hewitt, T. E., Wold, S., and Joiner, B. (1975). *In* "Quality Control in Laboratory Medicine" (J. B. Henry and J. Geigel, eds.), pp. 141–148. Masson Publ. Co., New York.

Westgard, J. O., Carey, R. N., Feldbruegge, D. H., and Jenkins, L. M. (1976). *Clin. Chem.* **22**, 489–496.

Westgard, J. O., de Vos, D. J., Hunt, M. R., Quam, E. F., Carey, R. N., and Garber, C. C. (1978a). *Am. J. Med. Technol.* **44**, 290–300.

Westgard, J. E., de Vos, D. J., Hunt, M. R., Quam, E. F., Carey, R. N., and Garber, C. C. (1978b). *Am. J. Med. Technol.* **44**, 420–430.

Westgard, J. E., de Vos, D. J., Hunt, M. R., Quam, E. F., Carey, R. N., and Garber, C. C. (1978c). *Am. J. Med. Technol.* **44**, 552–571.

Westgard, J. E., de Vos, D. J., Hunt, M. R., Quam, E. F., Carey, R. N., and Garber, C. C. (1978d). *Am. J. Med. Technol.* **44,** 727–742.

WHO Technical Report Series (1975). Rep. 26th T.R.S. No 565, WHO Expert Committee on Biological Standardization, pp. 29–61.

Witherspoon, L. R. (1976). *In* "Continuing Education Lectures," pp. 15-1 to 15-15. Southeastern Chapter, Soc. Nucl. Med., Atlanta.

Young, D. S., Pestaner, L. C., and Gibberman, V. (1975). *Clin. Chem. (N.Y.)* **21,** 1D–432D.

Mathematics in Clinical Chemistry

WENDELL T. CARAWAY

This chapter is intended to present practical problems encountered in the clinical laboratory and to use them to illustrate principles and applications of clinical chemistry. It is assumed that the reader has a basic knowledge of calculations in analytical chemistry involving molarity, normality,

CLINICAL BIOCHEMISTRY
Contemporary Theories and Techniques, Vol. 1

dilutions, pH, Beer's law, and elementary statistics, which are well-covered elsewhere (Routh, 1976; Blankenship and Campbell, 1976; Remson and Ackermann, 1977; Martin et al., 1975). In this chapter, we hope to reason out logically the steps in problem solving.

I. MOLAR ABSORPTIVITY AND ABSORPTION COEFFICIENTS

A. Beer's Law

According to Beer's law,

$$A = abc$$

where A is absorbance, a is a constant called absorptivity, b is the light path, and c is concentration. Since A has no units, the units for a are $b^{-1}c^{-1}$. When b is 1 cm and c is 1 mole/liter, a is defined as the molar absorptivity and is indicated by the Greek letter epsilon (ϵ); hence, $A = \epsilon bc$, where ϵ is the calculated absorbance of a 1-M solution with a 1-cm light path.

Molar absorptivities are characteristic constants for substances showing well-defined absorption peaks under specified conditions. Thus, if a chloroform solution containing 5.00 mg/liter of pure bilirubin with a molecular weight of 584 was found to have an absorbance of 0.520 at 453 nm (1.00-cm light path), then the molar absorptivity for bilirubin can be calculated as follows:

Concentration of bilirubin = 5 mg/liter = 0.005 gm/liter

$$= \frac{0.005}{584} \text{ mole/liter} = 8.56 \times 10^{-6} \text{ mole/liter}$$

$$\epsilon = \frac{A}{bc} = \frac{0.520}{(1)(8.56 \times 10^{-6})} = 60,750$$

Similarly, if the molar absorptivity is known, the concentration of an unknown solution may be calculated. Thus, if a solution of bilirubin under the above conditions shows an absorbance of 0.486, the concentration is:

$$c = \frac{A}{\epsilon b} = \frac{0.486}{(60,750)(1)} = 8.00 \times 10^{-6} \text{ mole/liter}$$

$$8 \times 10^{-6} \times 584 = 4.67 \times 10^{-3} \text{ gm/liter} = 4.67 \text{ mg/liter}$$

Molar absorptivities may also be determined for bilirubin in serum or for derivatives of compounds under specified reaction conditions, e.g., azobilirubin.

B. Absorption Coefficients

For spectrophotometric studies of substances of unknown identity, such as commonly occurs in toxicology, it is customary to define absorptivity as $A_{1\,cm}^{1\%}$, i.e., the calculated absorbance of a 1% solution with a 1-cm light path. In this notation, $A_{1\,cm}^{1\%}$ is called the absorption coefficient (sometimes called the extinction coefficient, $E_{1\,cm}^1$). Such coefficients may be found in handbooks of toxicology (Sunshine, 1969; Kaye, 1970) and may be listed for substances in dilute acids, bases, or other solvents and for wavelengths at maximum and minimum absorbances. Such data are useful for identification purposes.

Some years ago, capsules containing a white powder were peddled on a college campus with the claim of helping students stay awake. The contents weighed about 50 mg. A portion was dissolved in 0.1 N HCl and scanned in the uv spectrophotometer with a 1-cm light path cuvet. A solution containing 0.001 gm/dl (0.001%) of the unknown showed an absorbance peak at 273 nm with $A_{max} = 0.470$ and an absorbance minimum at 245 nm with $A_{min} = 0.140$. From these data,

$$\max A_{1\,cm}^{1\%} = \frac{A}{bc} = 0.470/(1)(0.001) = 470 \text{ and } \min A_{1\,cm}^{1\%} = 140$$

Reference to handbooks suggested that the entire spectral curve and absorption coefficients coincided well with those of caffeine. Comparison with a reference standard confirmed that the contents of the capsule appeared to be pure caffeine. Each capsule contained about the same amount of caffeine as one-half cup of coffee! Unfortunately, toxicological examinations are rarely this simple.

C. The NAD–NADH System

The oxidized and reduced forms of the coenzyme nicotinamide adenine dinucleotide are abbreviated NAD and NADH, respectively. This coenzyme participates in a number of enzymatic reactions involving dehydrogenases as illustrated by the following example:

$$\text{L-Lactate} + \text{NAD}^+ \xrightleftharpoons{\text{LD}} \text{pyruvate} + \text{NADH} + \text{H}^+$$

where LD in this reaction is lactate dehydrogenase. At 340 nm, NADH exhibits maximum absorbance with $\epsilon = 6220$, whereas NAD shows no absorbance. This property permits the application of the system for the determination of lactate, pyruvate, or LD activity. Other enzyme reactions may be coupled so that the final step involves the appearance or disappearance of NADH.

1. Determination of Lactate

A typical procedure is as follows: add 2.0 ml of fresh whole blood to 4.0 ml of 8% (w/v) perchloric acid solution, mix, and centrifuge. Add 0.20 ml of supernatant to 2.8 ml of buffered solution containing excess NAD and LD. Incubate 30 min at 37°C and measure absorbance against a reagent blank at 340 nm in a cuvet with a 1-cm light path. Assume that the reaction goes to completion and that the observed absorbance is entirely due to NADH generated in the reaction. Calculate the blood lactate concentration.

The *dilution* of the blood sample in the final reaction mixture is

$$\frac{2.0}{6.0} \times \frac{0.2}{3.0} = \frac{0.4}{18.0}$$

The dilution *factor* is the reciprocal of the dilution = 18.0/0.4 = 45. To derive a calibration constant, assume that $A_{340} = 1.000$. The concentration of NADH in the final reaction mixture is

$$\frac{A}{\epsilon} = 1.000/6220 = 1.61 \times 10^{-4} \text{ mole/liter}$$

Each mole of lactate generates 1 mole of NADH. Therefore, the concentration of lactate in the original blood is $1.61 \times 10^{-4} \times 45 = 7.24 \times 10^{-3}$ mole/liter = 7.24 mmole/liter. For this method then,

$$A \times 7.24 = \text{blood lactate in mmole/liter}$$

To express as mg/dl, multiply mmole/liter by the molecular weight of lactic acid (90) to obtain mg/liter and divide by 10 to obtain mg/dl. $A \times 7.24 \times 90/10 = A \times 65.2 = $ blood lactate in mg/dl expressed as lactic acid.

2. Determination of Lactate Dehydrogenase

A typical procedure is as follows: To a cuvet with a 1-cm light path, add 2.5 ml of buffer, 0.2 ml of NADH solution, and 0.1 ml of serum. Incubate at constant temperature to destroy endogenous keto acids, then initiate the reaction by adding 0.2 ml of pyruvate solution. Record readings continuously or at timed intervals and calculate the decrease in absorbance per minute over a linear portion of the curve.

The dilution of serum is 0.1/3.0; the dilution factor is 30. Suppose

ΔA/min $= -0.040$. This corresponds to the disappearance of NADH in the final reaction mixture:

$0.04/6220 = 6.43 \times 10^{-6}$ mole/liter $= 6.43$ μmole/liter of solution/min

Multiplying by 30, the dilution factor, we obtain 193 μmoles of NADH/liter of serum in 1 min. Each mole of pyruvate requires 1 mole of NADH. Hence, we have 193 μmoles of pyruvate reacted per minute per liter of serum. International Units (U) of enzyme activity are equal to the number of micromoles of substrate utilized in 1 min; hence, the lactate dehydrogenase activity $= 193$ U/liter of serum. In the same way, a change in absorbance (ΔA) of 1.00/minute can be shown to be equivalent to 4823 U/liter of serum or ΔA/min $\times 4823 =$ U/liter of serum.

II. UNITS OF ENZYME ACTIVITY

As noted above, 1 U (international unit) of enzyme activity is defined as the transformation of 1 μmole of substrate per minute. Bowers and Mc-Comb (1970) discuss this unit in more detail. Specific activity of an enzyme may be expressed in units per volume of body fluid as U/liter, U/ml, mU/ml, etc., to provide convenient units. This definition brings some semblance of uniformity to units of enzyme activity. However, reaction conditions must still be defined such as nature of substrate, buffer, temperature, pH, and so on. In other words, international units for different procedures are not interchangable.

To convert from older conventional units to international units, conversion is made so that the reaction is expressed in μmoles per minute. In the Shinowara *et al.* (1942) method of alkaline phosphatase, 1 U of enzyme activity was defined as the liberation of 1 mg of inorganic phosphorus (as phosphate) from β-glycerophosphate by 100 ml of serum in 60 min incubation time. The atomic weight of phosphorus is 31. Convert mg of P to μmoles, time to 1 min, and volume of serum to 1 liter.

1 SJR unit $= 1$ mg P/60 min/100 ml serum

$$= \frac{1 \text{ mg}}{31 \text{ mg/mmole}} \times \frac{1000 \text{ }\mu\text{mole}}{1 \text{ mmole}} \times \frac{1 \text{ min}}{60 \text{ min}} \times \frac{1000 \text{ ml}}{100 \text{ ml}}$$

$$= 5.4 \text{ U/liter}$$

Therefore, U $=$ SJR units $\times 5.4$.

When the substrate is not well-defined, such as the use of starch in a method for amylase activity, units are expressed in terms of products formed, e.g., as reducing sugars compared to micromoles of glucose.

The enzyme units for the SI system (Système International) are based on moles per second, rather than micromoles per minute. The unit of enzyme activity corresponding to the conversion of 1 mole per sec of substrate is called the *katal*. To convert U (μmole/min) to katal (mole/sec) multiply micromoles by 10^{-6} to obtain moles and divide minutes by 60 to obtain seconds.

$$1 \text{ U} = 1 \ \mu\text{mole/min} = \frac{1 \times 10^{-6}}{60} \text{ mole/sec} = 16.67 \times 10^{-9} \text{ katal}$$

Since 10^{-9} katal = 1 nanokatal, I U = 16.67 nanokatals (nkat). Hence, any enzyme activity expressed in international units may be converted to nanokatals by multiplying by 16.67. The liter is used as the standard volume, and enzyme activity is expressed as μkat, nkat, pkat, etc., per liter to obtain convenient units.

III. ABSORBANCE AT MULTIPLE WAVELENGTHS

A. Absorbance at Two Wavelengths

1. Two Chemical Forms with an Isosbestic Point

Equimolar concentrations of hemoglobin (Hb) and oxyhemoglobin (HbO$_2$) have equal absorbance at 805 nm, the isosbestic point for this system. At 650 nm, the ratio of absorbance, $R = A_{650}/A_{805}$, is approximately 4.45 for Hb and 0.43 for HbO$_2$ (Polanyi and Hehir, 1960). Once these ratios are established, the percent oxygen saturation for a mixture of the two forms may be obtained by interpolation between the two ratios. Thus, if a blood sample shows a ratio of 1.30,

$$\text{Percent O}_2 \text{ saturation} = \frac{4.45 - 1.30}{4.45 - 0.43} \times 100 = 78\%$$

The high absorbance of hemolyzed whole blood requires the use of cuvets with narrow light path. An alternate technique is to reflect light from the surface of whole blood, split the beam into two components, and measure the ratio of light passed through interference filters at 805 and 660 nm, respectively. The ratio of light reflected at 660 nm to light reflected at 805 nm is linearly related to oxygen saturation as in absorption measurements but with opposite slope.

Use of isosbestic points can be applied to determine relative concentrations of acid–base forms of indicators, NAD-NADH, and carboxyhemoglobin in the presence of oxyhemoglobin (Amenta, 1963).

2. Correction for Baseline Absorbance

In some applications, absorbance is measured at two wavelengths to partially correct for background absorbance contributed by extraneous color or turbidity unrelated to the substance of interest. In one automatic analyzer, for example, albumin is determined by a bromcresol green dye binding technique, which produces maximum absorbance at 600 nm. A second reading is taken at 540 nm to serve as a reference point, and the difference ($A_{600} - A_{540}$) is assumed to be proportional to the concentration of albumin. If the specimen is slightly hemolyzed, results would be falsely low since the absorbance of hemoglobin is about 6 times greater at 540 nm than at 600 nm. Lipemia would also result in lower values since light scattering (and apparent absorbance) is greater at the lower wavelength (see Section III, C).

B. The Allen Correction

If background absorbance can be shown to be linear, corrections can be made more accurately by taking readings at three wavelengths, two of which are removed from the point of maximum absorbance. This approach is referred to as the "baseline" technique or Allen correction (Allen, 1950; Allen and Rieman, 1953). In a method for measuring urinary estriol in late pregnancy, the final extract shows maximum absorbance at 525 nm. Readings are taken at 490 and 560 nm, averaged, and subtracted from the reading at 525 nm to give a corrected absorbance. Standards are processed in the same way. Typical curves for pregnancy and nonpregnancy urine specimens are shown in Fig. 1. The corrected absorbance is calculated as follows:

$$A_{corr} = A_{525} - \left(\frac{A_{490} + A_{560}}{2}\right)$$

This approach is useful in many spectrophotometric analyses provided that the background absorbance can be shown to be essentially *linear* over the range of wavelengths chosen.

The two background readings do not have to be taken at wavelengths equidistant from the peak (λ_x) nor must they necessarily be on opposite sides of the peak. When the wavelengths (λ) are not equidistant from λ_x, the corrected absorbance is obtained as follows where subscripts refer to corresponding wavelengths and absorbance readings:

$$A_{corr} = A_x - A_2 + \frac{\lambda_x - \lambda_2}{\lambda_1 - \lambda_2}(A_2 - A_1)$$

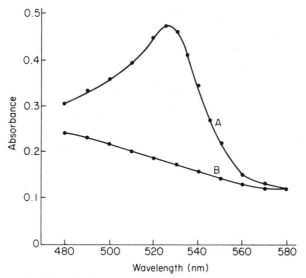

Fig. 1. Example of an Allen correction applied to determination of urinary estriol. Curve A, same urine with 15 mg/liter of added estriol. Curve B, nonpregnancy urine.

C. Correction for Light Scattering

When light is passed through a turbid solution, such as might occur in the presence of lipemic serum, some of the light is scattered (i.e., reflected or refracted) and fails to reach the photocell. This results in an apparent increase in absorbance, and this increase is greater at lower wavelengths. Assuming no other absorbing substances are present, a plot of log A versus log λ produces a straight line over most of the visible portion of the spectrum (Gaebler, 1943). In general,

$$A = k\lambda^b \tag{1}$$

$$\text{Log } A = \log k + b \log \lambda \tag{2}$$

The slope of the straight line, b, will be reasonably constant for a particular spectrophotometer for a given type of turbid system. In some applications, a reading of absorbance related to turbidity may be taken at a wavelength (say 700 nm), where serum components or reagents do not absorb appreciably. The contribution to absorbance at other wavelengths may then be estimated graphically or analytically.

A sample of grossly lipemic serum was diluted with saline solution and read against saline in a Beckman DBG spectrophotometer with 1-cm light

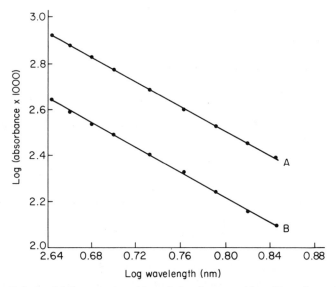

Fig. 2. Relationship between logarithm of absorbance and logarithm of wavelength on turbid solutions. Grossly lipemic serum was diluted 1:100 (A) and 1:200 (B) with 0.9% sodium chloride. Beckman DBG spectrophotometer.

path to produce the curves shown in Fig. 2. The slope of the parallel lines is -2.70. The ratio of absorbance for any two wavelengths will be

$$\frac{A_1}{A_2} = \frac{k\lambda_1^b}{k\lambda_2^b} = \left(\frac{\lambda_1}{\lambda_2}\right)^b$$

and

$$\text{Log}\,\frac{A_1}{A_2} = b\,\log\frac{\lambda_1}{\lambda_2}$$

Thus, if $\lambda_2 = 700$ nm and $b = -2.7$, then the absorbance A_1 due to turbidity at λ_1 (say 550 nm) can be calculated:

$$\text{Log}\,\frac{A_1}{A_2} = -2.7\,\log\frac{550}{700} = 0.2827$$

$$\frac{A_1}{A_2} = 1.92 \text{ or } A_1 = 1.92\,A_2$$

This type of correction has found application in direct spectrophotometric methods for bilirubin (Fog, 1958), hemoglobin (Shinowara, 1954), and sulfobromophthalein (BSP) in plasma or serum (Gaebler, 1945).

IV. THE HENDERSON–HASSELBALCH EQUATION

A. Buffers and pH

The ionization of a weak acid:

$$HA \xrightleftharpoons{K_a} H^+ + A^-$$

forms a buffer pair where K_a is the ionization constant and concentrations are expressed in moles/liter.

$$K_a = \frac{[H^+][A^-]}{[HA)]}$$

From this equation is derived the Henderson–Hasselbalch equation:

$$pH = pK_a + \log \frac{[A^-]}{[HA]} \tag{3}$$

where $pH = -\log [H^+]$ and $pK_a = -\log K_a$. Since K_a is influenced by concentrations of buffer, ionic strength, temperature, etc., the expression pK_a' is used in a particular situation.

Of the two species, HA is the proton donor and A^- is the proton acceptor. For weak bases [B] we may continue to use pK_a and substitute B for A^- and BH^+ for HA, respectively. Note that when $(A^-) = (HA)$, pH equals pK_a; when $\frac{[A^-]}{[HA]} = 10/1$, pH equals $pK_a + 1$; and when $\frac{[A^-]}{[HA]} = 1/10$, pH equals $pK_a - 1$. At $pK_a + 1$, we have 10/11 or 91% of the buffer in the form of A^-. At $pK_a + 1$, we have 1/11 or 9% of the buffer in the form of A^-. Hence, the effective range of a buffer system is about 2 pH units, i.e., $pK_a \pm 1$.

pK_a is usually known and problems involve estimation of pH from molar concentrations of A^- and HA or, conversely, estimating the concentrations of A^- (salt form) and HA (acid form) to produce a buffer of a given pH.

Example: Calculate the concentrations of sodium acetate and acetic acid required to prepare 0.1 M buffer with pH = 5.2.

$$K_a = 1.8 \times 10^{-5}, \text{ whence } pK_a = 5 - \log 1.8 = 4.75$$

By Eq. (3):

$$5.2 = 4.75 + \log \frac{[salt]}{[acid]}$$

$$\frac{[Salt]}{[Acid]} = \text{antilog } (5.2 - 4.75) = \frac{2.82}{1.00}$$

The sum of the relative concentrations of both forms is 3.82, i.e., 2.82 + 1.00, in the 0.1 M buffer. Therefore,

$$[\text{Salt}] = \frac{2.82}{3.82} \times 0.1 = 0.074 \ M$$

$$[\text{Acid}] = 0.100 - 0.074 = 0.026 \ M$$

Check: $\quad$ pH = $4.75 + \log \dfrac{0.074}{0.026} = 5.2.$

A system with more than one pK_a may be treated as above if the second pK is more than 2 pH units from the one of interest. This situation holds with phosphate buffer near pH 7, where $A^- = HPO_4^{2-}$, and $HA = H_2PO_4^-$, and pK_{a2}' is approximately 6.8. For dibasic acids, e.g. succinic acid with pK_{a1} is 4.21 and pK_{a2} is 5.65, the relative concentrations of the three forms at a given pH are obtained by applying the Henderson–Hasselbalch equation separately for each pK. Thus, at pH 4.90, we have:

$$4.90 = 4.21 + \log \frac{[HA^-]}{[H_2A]}$$

and

$$4.90 = 5.65 + \log \frac{[A^{2-}]}{[HA^-]}$$

from which the relative molar proportions of each form may be calculated.

B. Blood pH, Bicarbonate, and pCO$_2$

The carbonic acid–bicarbonate buffer system also participates in a second equilibrium system with water and dissolved carbon dioxide:

$$CO_2 + H_2O \overset{K_1}{\rightleftharpoons} H_2CO_3 \overset{K_2}{\rightleftharpoons} H^+ + HCO_3^-$$

Combination of the two equilibrium constants results in a single K'. For blood plasma at 37°C, the normal mean value of pK' is 6.10. Hence,

$$pH = 6.10 + \log \frac{[HCO_3^-]}{[H_2CO_3]} \tag{4}$$

With this value for pK', $[H_2CO_3]$ represents the sum of carbonic acid and dissolved CO_2 in equilibrium with the partial pressure of CO_2 in the gas phase. These are related by Henry's law: $[H_2CO_3] = \alpha pCO_2$. The mean value of α for normal plasma at 37°C is 0.0306 mmole $\times$ liter^{-1} $\times$ mm

Hg^{-1}. The Henderson–Hasselbalch equation may then be rewritten:

$$pH = 6.10 + \log [(HCO_3^-)]/0.03 \, pCO_2 \qquad (5)$$

This equation contains three unknowns and is determined uniquely if any two are known. In blood gas determinations, pH and pCO_2 are measured directly and bicarbonate is calculated. Note also that the total CO_2 content $= [HCO_3^-] + [H_2CO_3]$. Therefore, we may substitute (total CO_2 content $- 0.03 \, pCO_2$) for $[HCO_3^-]$ in the above equation.

Example: An arterial blood specimen at 37°C has a pH of 7.35 and pCO_2 of 50 mm Hg. Calculate bicarbonate and total CO_2 content. From Eq. (5):

$$7.35 = 6.10 + \log \frac{[HCO_3^-]}{(0.03)(50)}$$

$$\text{Log} \frac{[HCO_3^-]}{1.5} = 7.35 - 6.10 = 1.25$$

$$\frac{[HCO_3^-]}{1.5} = \text{antilog } 1.25 = 17.8$$

$$[HCO_3^-] = 26.7 \text{ mmole/liter}$$

$$\text{Total } CO_2 \text{ content} = [HCO_3^-] + [H_2CO_3] = 26.7 + (0.03)(50)$$

$$= 28.2 \text{ mmole/liter.}$$

Natelson and Nobel (1977) have pointed out that pK' in plasma of critically ill patients can vary significantly from the normal mean value of 6.10. If we substitute $pK' = 6.00$ in the above example we find $[HCO_3^-] = 33.6$ mmole/liter rather than 26.7. Thus, small changes in pK' or errors in measuring pH introduce significant errors in calculated values when we take the antilog of $(pH - pK')$.

V. OSMOLALITY

A. Osmolality of Pure Solutions

The osmolality of an aqueous solution is defined as the sum of the number of moles of all dissolved ions and undissociated molecules in 1 kg of water. Results are expressed in Osmole/kg or mOsmole/kg. A solution containing 1 Osmole/kg has a freezing point of $-1.86°C$. Hence, osmolality may be determined directly by measuring the depression of the freezing point.

If we dissolve 1 mole (180 gm) of glucose in 1 kg of water, we should have a solution containing 1 Osmole/kg since glucose does not dissociate into ions. The observed freezing point depression, obtained from a Handbook of Chemistry and Physics, is close to 1.86°C. In fact, it is slightly greater than expected because of hydration of the glucose molecule.

If we dissolve 1 mole (58.45 gm) of sodium chloride in 1 kg of water, we should expect the solution to contain 2 Osmole/kg since the sodium chloride dissociates into two ions. The actual value is somewhat less because of some association of Na^+Cl^-. The term "osmotic coefficient" is introduced to correct for this deviation from ideal behavior. The osmotic coefficient of NaCl is a function of concentration and varies between 0.91 and 0.95 for concentrations ranging from 0.05 to 1.1 molal. A value of 0.93 is used for most clinical analyses. A solution containing 9.00 gm of NaCl per liter of solution contains 9.040 gm NaCl per kg of water (data from Handbooks). From this, we can calculate the osmolality to be:

$$\frac{9.040}{58.45} \times 2 \times 0.93 \times 1000 = 288 \text{ mOsmole/kg}$$

The observed freezing point depression is 0.534°C corresponding to an osmolality of $0.534/1.86 \times 1000 = 287$ mOsmole/kg.

B. Serum Osmolality

The major contributions to serum osmolality come from sodium ions and matching monovalent ions, principally chloride and bicarbonate. Proteins, because of their high molecular weight, contribute almost nothing to serum osmolality. Thus, osmolality of serum is essentially identical with that of glomerular filtrate. If we ignore small differences between osmolality and molarity for concentrations found in serum, the contribution to osmolality from sodium and its matching ions is:

$$\text{mOsmole/kg} = Na^+ \text{ (mmole/liter)} \times 2 \times 0.93 = 1.86 \times Na^+$$

For glucose,

$$\text{mOsmole/kg} = \frac{\text{glucose (mg/dl)} \times 10}{180} = \text{glucose}/18$$

For urea, expressed as urea nitrogen in mg/dl, the molecular weight of two nitrogens = 28:

$$\text{mOsmole/kg} = \text{urea N (mg/dl)} \times 10/28 = \frac{\text{urea N}}{2.8}$$

Another 9 mOsmole/kg is added to account for other molecules and ions normally present. The complete equation, as proposed by Dorwart and

Chalmers (1975) is:

Serum osmolality, mOsmole/kg = 1.86Na + glucose/18   (6)

$$+ \text{ urea } N/2.8 + 9$$

A rapid approximation can be obtained from the equation:

$$\text{mOsmole/kg} = 2 \times Na + \text{glucose}/20 + \text{urea } N/3 \qquad (7)$$

Since osmolality is based on solute per kilogram of water, the results are independent of space occupying substances. A serum, for example, might contain as much as 10 gm/dl of triglycerides. This would decrease the apparent serum sodium by about 10%, measured as mmole/liter, but would have no significant effect on osmolality. A similar situation occurs with unusually high concentrations of serum protein, such as in patients with multiple myeloma.

VI. RENAL CLEARANCE

A. General Equation

Assume a patient with a plasma creatinine of 1.0 mg/dl and urine creatinine of 100 mg/dl. This means that each ml of urine contains the same amount of creatinine that is present in 100 ml of plasma. If the urine output is 1 ml/min then, in effect, we are removing or "clearing" the creatinine from 100 ml of plasma each minute. Hence,

$$\text{Renal clearance } (C), \text{ ml/min} = \frac{U}{P} \times V$$

where U is the concentration of substance in urine; P is the concentration of substance in plasma; and V is the urine excretion in ml/minute. Criteria for accurate results include careful collection of a timed urine specimen, constant concentrations in plasma during the period of urine collection, and accurate measurement of U and P. There is some evidence that plasma creatinine concentration alone is superior to creatinine clearance as a test of glomerular function (Morgan et al., 1978).

Renal clearance is customarily corrected to an average body surface area of 1.73 m² by multiplying by 1.73/A where A is body surface area in m². Values for A may be obtained from nomograms or by use of the equation

$$A = 0.007184 \ W^{0.425} \ H^{0.725} \qquad (8)$$

or $\log A = 0.425 \log W + 0.725 \log H - 2.144$ (9)

where W is the body weight in kg and H is the height in cm.

DuBois and DuBois (1916) derived the above equation from direct measurements on a small number of individuals. They also showed that a simpler equation could be used with an average error of only 2.2%, that is,

$$A = 0.01672 \sqrt{W \times H} \tag{10}$$

Example: A patient with height 172 cm and weight 75 kg has a plasma creatinine of 1.2 mg/dl. A 24-hour urine collection measures 1250 ml and has a creatinine concentration of 150 mg/dl. Calculate creatinine clearance as ml/min corrected for surface area.

$$C = \frac{UCr}{PCr} \times V \times \frac{1.73}{A}$$

$$V = \frac{1250}{60 \times 24} = 0.868 \text{ ml/min}$$

$$A = 0.01672 \sqrt{75 \times 172} = 1.90 \text{ m}^2$$

$$C = \frac{150}{1.2} \times 0.868 \times \frac{1.73}{1.90} = 99 \text{ ml/min}$$

Correction for A is inadequate in infants up to 6 months old since they have a higher percent total body water, hence relatively lower lean body mass (McCance and Widdowson, 1952). Plasma creatinine remains fairly constant between ages 20 and 80 years; however, creatinine clearance falls about 50% during this age interval. This apparent anomaly is explained by a fall in creatinine production, which is proportionately similar to the fall in creatinine clearance (Morgan *et al.*, 1978).

B. Ratio of Clearances

Renal clearance of a substance may also be expressed as a ratio of creatinine clearance. This eliminates the need for a timed specimen, a major pitfall in measuring clearance alone. Parathyroid hormone, for example, inhibits the tubular reabsorption of phosphate resulting in an increased clearance of phosphate. Expressed as a ratio,

$$\frac{C_{\text{phosphate}}}{C_{\text{creatinine}}} = \frac{\dfrac{UP}{PP} \times V}{\dfrac{UCr}{PCr} \times V} = \frac{UP \times PCr}{PP \times UCr}$$

This ratio is normally 0.07 to 0.23 but is reported to range from 0.21 to 0.57 in patients with hyperparathyroidism (Reiss and Alexander, 1959).

The ratio of the renal clearance of amylase to creatinine has been proposed to distinguish acute pancreatitis from all other causes of hyperamylasemia (Warshaw and Fuller, 1975). Analogous to the example for phosphate,

$$\frac{CAm}{CCr}(\%) = \frac{UAm \times PCr}{PAm \times UCr} \times 100$$

The ratios so obtained, however, have been shown to be method dependent (Levitt *et al.*, 1977). By a saccharogenic method, mean ratios rose from 2.19% in normals to 6.57% in patients with acute pancreatitis.

VII. DISTRIBUTION BETWEEN SOLVENTS

Consider a substance A dissolved in two solvents that are immiscible and are in contact. When equilibrium is established by mixing, the ratio of the *concentrations* of A in the two phases will be constant and

$$\frac{C_1}{C_2} = K$$

where K is called the *distribution coefficient*. For clinical work, we usually consider C_1 the concentration in the organic phase and C_2 the concentration in the aqueous phase. The relative *amounts* or weights of the substance in each phase will also depend on the volumes of the phases since amount = concentration × volume.

$$w_1 = C_1V_1 = \text{weight in solvent phase with volume } V_1$$

$$w_2 = C_2V_2 = \text{weight in aqueous phase with volume } V_2$$

Dividing

$$\frac{w_1}{w_2} = \frac{C_1V_1}{C_2V_2} = K \cdot \frac{V_1}{V_2}$$

The percent extracted into phase 1 will be:

$$E = \frac{C_1V_1}{C_1V_1 + C_2V_2} \times 100$$

Dividing both numerator and denominator by C_2V_1,

$$E = \frac{100\,K}{K + V_2/V_1} \tag{11}$$

Example: The solubility of phenobarbital is given as 25 mg/ml in chloroform (C_1) and 1.0 mg/ml in water (C_2). The expected value for K is 25. If the two phases have equal volumes,

$$E = \frac{100\ K}{K + 1} = \frac{(100)(25)}{26} = 96.2\%$$

Consider two extractions where the volume of chloroform in each case is one-half the aqueous phase, that is, $V_2/V_1 = 2/1$.

$$E = \frac{100\ K}{K + 2} = 92.6\%$$

which leaves 7.4% in the aqueous phase. The second extraction will remove 92.6% of the remaining 7.4% or 6.9% for a total extraction of 99.5%. Thus, greater efficiency is obtained by multiple extractions for a given total volume of solvent.

Since the pK_a of phenobarbital is 7.3, the fraction of dissociated anion in the aqueous phase is very small and is ignored in the above example. If the solution is buffered at pH 7.3, one-half of the total concentration would be in the ionized form, i.e., the fraction ionized (α) = 0.50. In this event,

$$\frac{C_1}{C_2(1 - \alpha)} = K \quad \text{and} \quad E = \frac{100\ K\ (1 - \alpha)}{K + V_2/V_1}$$

Again consider that the two phases have equal volume. Then,

$$E = \frac{(100)(25)(0.5)}{25 + 1} = 48.1\%$$

This leaves 51.9% in the aqueous phase.

In the above example, the anionic form is assumed to be insoluble in chloroform. For a given pH and pK_a, the value of α is readily calculated by using the Henderson–Hasselbalch equation.

Example: Assume that 3.0 ml of serum containing theophylline ($pK_a = 8.8$) is buffered at pH 7.4 and extracted with two 50-ml volumes of chloroform. The solubility of theophylline is approximately 8.3 mg/ml in water and 9.1 mg/ml in chloroform. Estimate percent extracted.

$$K = 9.1/8.3 = 1.10$$

By the Henderson–Hasselbalch equation:

$$7.4 = 8.8 + \log \frac{\alpha}{1 - \alpha}$$

whence $\alpha = 0.0383$ and $(1 - \alpha) = 0.9617$. For the first extraction,

$$E = \frac{(100)(1.10)(0.9617)}{1.10 + 3/50} = 91.2\%$$

For the second extraction:

$$(0.912)(100 - 91.2) = 8.0\%$$

Total extracted: $91.2 + 8.0 = 99.2\%$.

Jatlow (1975) used 3 ml of serum + 2ml of phosphate buffer, pH 7.4, and a single extraction with 30 ml of chloroform–isopropyl alcohol (95/5). Experimentally, starting with 5 ml of water, one finds that the final aqueous phase is 5.5 ml; hence we could expect

$$E = \frac{(100)(1.10)(0.9617)}{1.10 + 5.5/29.5} = 82.2\%$$

This compares favorably with the reported recovery of 84.9% after back extraction into 0.1 M NaOH.

In the case of weak bases, the base form, B, is usually more soluble in organic solvents than the acid form BH^+. Morphine, for example, with $pK_a = 9.85$, is extracted into chloroform from alkaline solution with a distribution coefficient of 4.1. For weak bases, α is the fraction corresponding to B and

$$E = \frac{100 \, K \, \alpha}{K + V_2/V_1} \tag{12}$$

We may also estimate V_2/V_1 to obtain a desired extraction efficiency. For morphine, a 98% extraction efficiency by chloroform from alkaline solution corresponds to

$$98 = \frac{(100)(4.1)}{4.1 + V_2/V_1}$$

from which $V_2/V_1 = 1/12$. Hence, we would use 12 volumes of chloroform to 1 volume of aqueous solution to obtain 98% extraction of morphine.

In general, it is more efficient to acidify samples to extract weak acids and to alkalinize to extract weak bases.

VIII. COMPLEX ANALYTICAL PROCEDURES

Some procedures require use of multiple steps, extractions, and aliquots that tend to complicate calculation of final results. Ideally, a single constant can be derived to simplify calculations. Thus, one follows through a multistep procedure to arrive at a simple factor for calculation of final results.

Example: In a procedure for the quantitative determination of urobilinogen, 50 ml of urine is mixed with 25 ml of ferrous sulfate solution
and 25 ml of sodium hydroxide solution. The mixture is filtered after 1
hour. To 30 ml of filtrate is added 3 ml of acetic acid and 20 ml of petro-
leum ether. After extraction, 5 ml of the ether layer is mixed with 5 ml of
Ehrlich's reagent (aqueous) and 10 ml of saturated sodium acetate solution. The solution is extracted again, and the absorbance is measured on
the lower aqueous phase. A standard, containing phenol red in alkaline
solution, is equivalent in color to 3.46 mg of urobilinogen per liter of final
colored solution measured in the test. Derive a factor such that

$$\frac{A_u}{A_s} \times \text{factor} = \text{mg urobilinogen/liter of urine}$$

where A_u = absorbance of the unknown and A_s = absorbance of the
standard.

Rationale: If a standard containing a known concentration of urobilinogen had been carried through the entire procedure,

$$\frac{A_u}{A_s} \times C_s = C_{u'}$$

where C_s = concentration of the standard and C_u = concentration of the
unknown. Since it was not, we need to know the extent of dilution of the
original sample. Follow through the procedure to determine the volume of
urine that contained the urobilinogen present in the final 15 ml of aqueous
solution.

1. 50 ml of urine + 2 reagents (25 ml each) = 100 ml of mixture containing 50 ml of urine.
2. Use 30-ml filtrate. $30/100 \times 50 = 15$ ml of urine.
3. Extract 30-ml filtrate with 20 ml of ether = 15 ml of urine.
4. Use 5 ml ether phase. $5/20 \times 15 = 3.75$ ml of urine.
5. Extract 5 ml ether phase with 15 ml final aqueous solution =
   3.75 ml of urine in 15 ml of final solution.
6. $15/3.75 = 4$-fold dilution of urine in final solution.
7. Concentration of standard = 3.46 mg/liter.
8. $\dfrac{A_u}{A_s} \times 3.46 \times 4 = \dfrac{A_u}{A_s} \times 13.84 = $ mg urobilinogen/liter of urine.

An alternate and simpler procedure would be to obtain the product of
all dilution factors in the procedure. These are found in steps 1, 3, and 5 to
be 100/50, 20/30, and 15/5, respectively. The dilution factor is 100/50 ×
20/30 × 15/5 = 4 as found in step 6. In case of doubt, it is better to proceed through each step as shown in the more detailed example.

IX. EXPONENTIAL FUNCTIONS AND HALF-LIFE

A number of situations arise where a substance disappears at a rate proportional to the amount present at any point in time. This applies to the rate of decay of radioisotopes. Similar kinetics may apply to the rate of elimination of drugs, BSP clearance from plasma, red blood cell survival, and the decrease in blood glucose during an intravenous glucose tolerance test.

The rate of decay for a radioisotope is given by the differential equation:

$$\frac{-dA}{dt} = \lambda A$$

where A is radioactivity, t is time, and λ is rate of decay. Integrating between limits with activity A_0 at the time zero (t_0) we obtain:

$$\ln \frac{A}{A_0} = -\lambda t$$

where ln refers to natural or Naperian logarithms with base e. The time required for activity to drop to one-half the original activity is called the half-life $(t_{1/2})$. At this time,

$$\frac{A}{A_0} = \tfrac{1}{2} \qquad \text{and} \qquad \ln \tfrac{1}{2} = -\lambda t_{1/2} \tag{13}$$

$$\lambda = \frac{\ln 2}{t_{1/2}} = \frac{0.693}{t_{1/2}}$$

When the half-life is known, λ may be calculated and used to determine relative activity at any other time.

Example: The half-life for ^{51}Cr is 27.8 days. Find the percent of activity remaining 12 days after the date of assay. By Eq. (13),

$$\lambda = 0.693/27.8 = 0.025 \text{ day}^{-1}$$

Let A_0 be 100% at time t_0.

$$\ln \frac{A}{100} = -(0.025)(12) = -0.300$$

From a table of natural logarithms,

$$\frac{A}{100} = 0.741 \text{ or } A = 74.1\%$$

To use log tables with base 10, we note that $\ln x = 2.303 \log_{10} x$.

$$2.303 \log \frac{A}{A_0} = -\lambda t \quad \text{or} \quad \log \frac{A}{A_0} = -0.434\,\lambda t$$

Hence,

$$\log \frac{A}{100} = -(0.434)(0.025)(12) = -0.1302$$

$$\frac{A}{100} = 0.741 \text{ (as above)}$$

When radioisotope assays are postdated, assign a negative value to t. In the above example the activity at 12 days before t_0 can be calculated:

$$\log \frac{A}{100} = (-0.434)(0.025)(-12) = 0.1302$$

$$\frac{A}{100} = 1.35 \text{ or } A = 135\%$$

In practice, it is convenient to use semilog paper with activity plotted on the log scale versus time on the linear scale. A straight line is drawn between (A_{100}, t_0) and $(A_{50}, t_{1/2})$. This line may be extrapolated in either

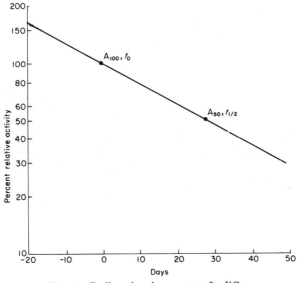

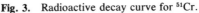

Fig. 3. Radioactive decay curve for ^{51}Cr.

direction to provide relative values for A at any time before or after t_0 (Fig. 3).

Intravenous glucose tolerance tests have been evaluated in terms of a constant, K, defined as the rate of disappearance of glucose from the blood, expressed as percent per minute of the 10-min level. Values for blood glucose are plotted versus time in minutes. The time required for the glucose level to fall to one-half the 10-min level = $t_{1/2}$.

$$\lambda = \frac{0.693}{t_{1/2}}$$

$$K = 100 \lambda = \frac{69.3}{t_{1/2}} \cong \frac{70}{t_{1/2}}$$

This equation is given in some textbooks without further explanation. Values for K are decreased in patients with diabetes compared to normal.

Nadeau (1954) proposed a somewhat similar velocity constant for the BSP test. Blood specimens were drawn at two time intervals following intravenous injection of BSP and the concentration or percent retention of BSP determined.

R_1 = percent retention at time t_1 (in minutes)

R_2 = percent retention at time t_2

$$K = \frac{\log R_1 - \log R_2}{t_2 - t_1}$$

Optimum times suggested for drawing specimens were 15 min and 30 min.

The concept of half-life is also useful in monitoring drug therapy. Depending on metabolic conversion or rate of excretion, patients with poor liver or kidney function may eliminate a drug more slowly (longer half-life) and require downward modification of dosage schedules. Children, on the other hand, tend to have decreased half-lives for some drugs compared to adults. The rate of elimination from the circulation may be biphasic, i.e., a rapid decrease in plasma levels as the drug enters the tissues, then a slower rate of decrease as the drug is eliminated from the tissues. A good example of the usefulness of pharmacokinetic studies is the work of Koch–Weser and Klein (1971) on the antiarrhythmic drug procainamide.

The concentration of a drug remaining after n half-lives is equal to $(0.5)^n$. After four half-lives, about 94% of the drug has been eliminated since $(0.5)^4 = 0.0625$, equivalent to about 6% of the drug remaining. The same calculation applies to decay of radioisotopes.

X. EMPIRICAL CURVE FITTING

Linear regression analysis by the method of least squares is used to determine the equation of the best straight line through a series of points. When data does not appear to follow a linear relationship, empirical equations are useful to approximate the curve. Such equations may or may not have any theoretical justification. Applications of empirical curve fitting include the use of programable calculators, microprocessors, and computers, as well as manual calculations.

A. Nonlinear Calibration Curves

Deviations from Beer's law tend to produce a parabolic curve when absorbance (A) is plotted against concentration (C). Two types of equations are generally used to obtain a curve to fit the data. One of these is:

$$C = \frac{aA}{1 + bA} \tag{14}$$

This can be rewritten as the equation of a straight line by taking reciprocals:

$$\frac{1}{C} = \frac{1}{a}\frac{1}{A} + \frac{b}{a} \tag{15}$$

where $1/a$ is the slope and b/a is the y intercept. Values for a and b may be obtained by graphing results or by linear regression analysis. It is *always* advisable to plot results to detect potential outliers that could grossly distort values obtained by simple linear regression.

Another equation describes a parabola where

$$C = aA + bA^2 \tag{16}$$

This is rewritten in linear form as

$$\frac{C}{A} = a + bA \tag{17}$$

where b is the slope and a is the y intercept. For Eq. (14) or (16), $C = 0$ when $A = 0$. When $b = 0$, the equations reduce simply to $C = aA$, that is, the equation for Beer's law at constant light path.

Example: A procedure for the direct determination of creatinine in serum involved color development with alkaline picrate, reading A_1 versus a reagent blank, then acidifying with a negligible volume of acetic acid and reading A_2. The difference in the two readings (A) was related to concentration of creatinine. Results obtained by a standard addition method, shown in Table I, were found not to follow Beer's law. Fitting the data to Eq. (14) by linear regression analysis of Eq. (15) resulted in

$$C = \frac{14.4 \, A}{1 - 0.294 \, A} \tag{18}$$

Fitting the data to Eq. (16) by linear regression analysis of Eq. (17) resulted in

$$C = 13.7 \, A + 7.0 \, A^2 \tag{19}$$

Equations (18) and (19) were then used to calculate C from observed values of A to determine which curve gave the best fit. From the results shown in Table I, it appears that either equation fits the data satisfactorily up to 10 mg/dl but that Eq. (19) provides a closer approach to the assigned standard values over the entire range.

The deviations from regression measure the failure of the line to fit the data. Let d = difference between assigned and calculated results. The sum of the squares of the deviations, Σd^2, is 0.92 for Eq. (18) and 0.38 for Eq. (19), thus confirming that the latter equation provides a better fit to the data over the entire range.

B. Data Reduction to Linear Form

As shown above, reduction of data to a linear equation facilitates calculation of constants from readings on standards which, in turn, permits calculation of results for unknowns. This principle is used in a variety of applications to data obtained by radioimmunoassay (RIA). In this tech-

TABLE I

Nonlinear Calibration Curve for Serum Creatinine

		Calculated C (mg/dl)	
C (mg/dl)	A	Eq. (18)	Eq. (19)
1.0	0.068	1.0	1.0
4.0	0.260	4.1	4.0
7.0	0.433	7.1	7.2
10.0	0.578	10.0	10.3
13.0	0.700	12.7	13.0
16.0	0.801	15.1	15.5
	Σd^2	0.92	0.38

TABLE II

Determination of Digoxin by Radioimmunoassay

			Calculated x		
x (ng/ml)	cpm	%B	Eq. (20)	Eq. (21)	Eq. (22)
0.0	13.520	100.0	0.02	0.02	0.01
0.4	10,816	80.0	0.39	0.40	0.39
1.0	8,316	61.5	0.96	0.97	0.96
2.0	5,684	42.0	2.07	2.09	2.09
3.0	4,546	33.6	2.96	2.96	2.97
5.0	3,098	22.9	5.01	4.95	4.98
		Σd^2	0.0087	0.0135	0.0112

nique, labeled and unlabeled antigen compete for binding sites on an antibody. After suitable equilibration, the bound and unbound (free) forms of the antigen are separated, and one or the other form of the labeled antigen is counted for radioactivity. For our purpose, we shall assume that the bound form (B) is counted. When no unlabeled antigen is present, $B =$

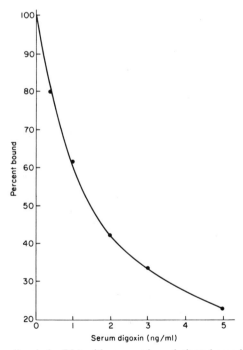

Fig. 4. Serum digoxin by RIA with percent bound plotted on a linear scale.

B_0. As the concentration or "dose" of unlabeled antigen (x) is increased, B will decrease in a nonlinear fashion. Typical results for a digoxin assay are listed in Table II and shown in Fig. 4. Counts per unit time may be plotted directly or converted to a percent of B_0, that is, $\%B = B/B_0 \times 100$.

Drawing the best curve through the points of Fig. 4 may be subject to considerable error. The curve can be "straightened out" to some extent by plotting on semilog paper (Fig. 5), and this may be adequate for visible interpolation. Since the original curve appears more or less hyperbolic, we could plot the reciprocal of the counts (or $100/\%B$) versus concentration to produce a curve approaching linearity for some assays (Fig. 6). For the data shown,

$$\frac{100}{\%B} = 0.985 + 0.675\,x \tag{20}$$

Calculated values for x and Σd^2 are shown in the table.

A more common approach, suitable for programable calculators, is to perform a logit–log transformation. This requires the use of a standard containing no unlabeled antigen in order to obtain a value for B_0.

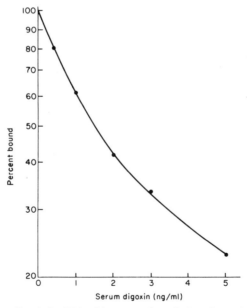

Fig. 5.   Serum digoxin by RIA with percent bound plotted on a logarithmic scale.

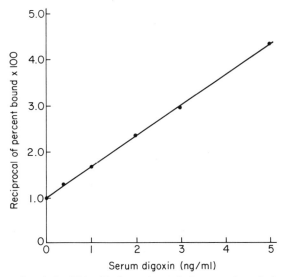

Fig. 6.   Serum digoxin by RIA with the reciprocal of percent bound plotted on a linear scale.

Let x equal the concentration of unlabeled antigen or "dose", and y equal $B/B_0 \times 100$:

$$\text{Logit } y = \log \frac{y}{100 - y}$$

$$\text{Logit } y = a + b \log x \tag{21}$$

$$x = \text{antilog} \left[\frac{\text{logit } y - a}{b} \right]$$

Equation (21) is readily solved by linear regression analysis. For the data shown, logit $y = 0.1915 - 1.034 \log x$. A plot of the data is shown in Fig. 7 and calculated values are given in Table II. The calculated value for zero concentration (B_0) is approximated by using $B = 99\%$.

C. Multiple Regression Analysis

Most equations considered thus far have involved a dependent variable (y) as a function of one independent variable (x) or $y = f(x)$. Cases arise when more than one independent variable contributes the value of y, that is, $y = f(x_1, x_2, x_3, \ldots x_n)$. The general equation for y becomes $y = a + b_1x_1 + b_2x_2 + b_3x_3 + \cdots b_nx_n$, etc. One example is given in

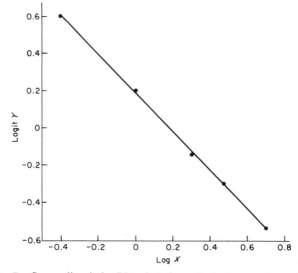

Fig. 7. Serum digoxin by RIA plotted as a logit–log transformation.

Section VI, Eq. (8) where body surface area is shown as a function of both weight and height. Solution of these equations is performed by multiple linear-regression analysis (see standard textbooks on statistics). The procedure is time-consuming if done manually; however, most programable calculators may be used for regression analyses for two or three independent variables. A few examples are given.

McKiel and Albertson (1978) proposed the following equation for handling radioimmunoassay data that is claimed to provide improved fit for unsaturated assays:

$$y = a + b_1 x + b_2 xy$$

where y = percent bound, $B/B_0 \times 100$, and x = standard dose. Here y appears on both sides of the equation but xy may be treated as one of the variables. Multiple regression analysis of the data in Table II results in

$$y = 100.5 - 0.681x - 0.651xy \tag{22}$$

Calculated values for x are shown in the table.

McLean and Hastings (1935) presented an equation for estimating ionized calcium in serum, based on the determination of total calcium and total protein. Calculations were cumbersome and a nomogram was devised to facilitate use of the equation. A simplified form of this equation is given by Zeisler (1954). By assuming values for total calcium and total protein over wide ranges, the corresponding concentration of ionized calcium may be calculated and such data used for regression analysis. When this was done the following equation was obtained:

Ionized Ca^{2+} (mg/dl) = 2.41 + 0.55 × total Ca (mg/dl)

$$- 0.47 \times TP \text{ (gm/dl)} \quad (23)$$

This equation provides values in reasonably good agreement with those predicted by the McLean–Hastings equation or nomogram. Such equations provide only approximations and are no substitute for direct measurements of ionized calcium by using ion-specific electrodes (Ladenson *et al*, 1978).

Various equations have also been proposed for predicting normal blood volumes from height and weight measurements or from surface areas which, in turn, were estimated from height and weight. Hidalgo (1962) derived the following for normal males and females where V = total blood volume in liters and SA = surface area in square meters.

$$\text{Males:} \quad V = 3.29 \times SA - 1.229 \quad (24)$$

$$\text{Females:} \quad V = 3.47 \times SA - 1.954 \quad (25)$$

Although these equations described their results satisfactorily for normal adults, the large residuals are mathematically unsatisfactory since V becomes zero whereas SA is still positive.

Surface areas and blood volumes were calculated from Eqs. (24) and (25) over a wide range of height (meters) and weight (kilograms) and fitted to the regression equation

$$V = aH^m W^n$$

by using $\log V = \log a + m \log H + n \log W$. The value for m was close to 1.0 and the value for n was between 0.5 and 0.6. To simplify calculations, the data were then fitted to $V = aHW^{0.5}$ to produce the following equations:

$$\text{Males:} \quad V = 0.330 \, HW^{0.5} \quad (26)$$

$$\text{Females:} \quad V = 0.300 \, HW^{0.5} \quad (27)$$

Values obtained with the latter equations showed close agreement with those obtained by Hidalgo's equations, and there is no residual volume as H and W approach zero. Similar values for the constants were obtained when the equation was applied to other raw data from the literature.

In a study of normal values, Goldberg *et al.* (1973) investigated the contribution of several demographic factors on serum concentrations of seven constituents in healthy subjects. Among these were age, sex, social class, body weight, and hypertension. Sexes were grouped separately and the effects of the four remaining variables on the test result were estimated by multiple regression analysis. For example, the following equations were derived to provide an estimate of normal serum uric acid in males and females. Results are expressed in mg/liter.

Males: mg/liter $= -0.122A + 0.118SC + 0.011\ BP$

$$+\ 0.131\ W + 42\ (\pm 20.2)$$

Females: mg/liter $= 0.19A + 0.158SC + 0.043\ BP$

$$+\ 0.163\ W + 11.6\ (\pm 18.7)$$

where A is age in years; SC is a social class rating ranging from 1 (highest) to 5 (lowest); BP is diastolic blood pressure in mm Hg; W is body weight in pounds. The values in parentheses at the end of the equations are the 95% confidence limits for the estimation. Such corrections for demographic variability seemed to improve the accuracy of each test in predicting underlying disease.

XI. STANDARD DEVIATION, STANDARD ERROR, AND STUDENT'S *t* TEST

Although this chapter is not designed to provide a background in statistics, a few useful and fundamental calculations will be described at this point. These are best illustrated by actual data.

Suppose that we analyze a given lot of control serum daily for a month and tabulate the results. If the analytical method is not subject to trend or shift during this period, we should expect only random errors to affect the results. Values would tend to group closely around the average or *mean* of the results, that is,

$$\bar{x} = \text{mean} = \frac{\Sigma x}{N}$$

where x is the individual values obtained over a 1-month period, Σx is the sum of these values, and N is number of values recorded.

We could next investigate the reproducibility of our determinations by noting how much each individual value deviates from the mean, that is, $(x - \bar{x})$. If we average up these deviations, taking the sign into account, the result should be zero. If we ignore the signs and obtain the average of the absolute values, the result is called the average deviation. The latter provides some indication of the reproducibility of results but is less convenient to handle statistically. For this purpose, we square the deviations, add them up, divide by the number of observations minus one, then take the square root. The result is called the standard deviation (s) and is expressed by

$$s = \sqrt{\frac{\Sigma(x - \bar{x})^2}{N - 1}}$$

The value ($N - 1$) is related to the number of "degrees of freedom" in statistical calculations. For practical purposes, results are about the same whether we use N or ($N - 1$) in the denominator, provided N is over 30.

The standard deviation is a measure of dispersal of values about the mean. A small s indicates that most values tend to cluster close to the mean and vice versa. For experiments involving repeated measurements on a single sample, results should show a frequency distribution curve described as a "normal" or Gaussian distribution as shown in Fig. 8. The total area under the curve represents 100% of the observed values.

The mean ± 1 s includes 68.27% of the values.

The mean ± 2 s includes 95.45% of the values.

The mean ± 3 s includes 99.73% of the values.

The mean ± 2 s is frequently used as the limits of acceptability for subsequent analyses. This range is also known as the 95% confidence limits since, by previous experience, this fraction of all results was found to fall within these limits. Results may still be expected to fall between ± 2 s and ± 3 s about 5% of the time (1 out of 20 determinations).

The *relative* standard deviation (RSD), also known as the coefficient of variation (CV), is equal to the standard deviation divided by the mean, that is, RSD = s/mean. This is usually expressed as percent RSD or CV and is intended to minimize the variation of the mean as it affects standard deviation. The wisdom of this approach is questionable. A CV of 10% on a serum creatinine of 1.0 mg/dl is only 0.1 mg/dl, a value within acceptable limits for clinical purposes. A CV of 10% on a serum sodium of 140 mmole/liter, however, is totally unacceptable.

A term known as standard deviation interval (SDI) has also been introduced by some quality control surveys. This value is the ratio of your deviation from the consensus mean compared to the standard deviation from the mean of all participants.

$$\text{SDI} = \frac{\text{your value} - \text{consensus mean}}{s \text{ of consensus mean}}$$

If the SDI is greater than 2.0, this means that your chances of being "off" from the consensus mean are greater than 95%.

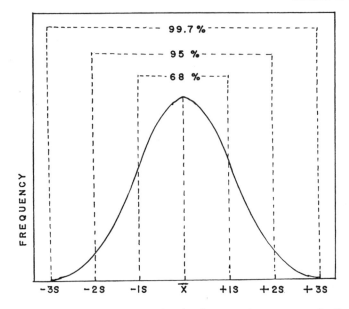

Fig. 8. Gaussian distribution curve showing the approximate areas under the curve for ±1, ±2, and ±3 standard deviations.

At this point a word of caution is advisable. The concept of standard deviation is strictly applicable only if the distribution of values is truly normal or Gaussian. Frequency distribution curves can be peaked, flat, skewed, or biphasic. Such distributions are not suitable for the usual mean and standard deviation approach. Mathematical transformations can often convert distributions to Gaussian forms suitable for further mathematical treatment.

If we continue to analyze the same control serum month after month, we find that the monthly means also form a normal distribution curve. From these data, we can calculate a new mean (the mean of the monthly means) and the standard deviation of the new mean. The standard deviation of the new mean, also called the *standard error,* can be predicted from the data for the first month by use of the relation:

$$SE = \frac{s}{\sqrt{N}}$$

where SE is the standard error of the mean, s is the standard deviation for a set of data (e.g., 1 month), N is the number of observations. Over a period of months, the means for each month should agree within ±2 SE 95% of the time. For example, a control serum analyzed for glucose daily for 30 days was found to have a mean value of 220 mg/dl with $s = 7$

TABLE III

Comparison of Serum Glucose Values by Two Methods[a]

Sample	Reference (mg/dl)	Proposed (mg/dl)	Difference (d)
1	52	56	+4
2	65	68	+3
3	80	83	+3
4	97	97	0
5	106	110	+4
6	115	121	+6
7	172	165	−7
8	203	210	+7
9	248	257	+9
10	311	308	−3

[a] $\Sigma d = +26$; $\bar{d}$ = difference between the means $= \dfrac{\Sigma d}{N} = \dfrac{26}{10} = 2.6$ mg/dl,

s_d = standard deviation of the differences $= \sqrt{\dfrac{\Sigma(d - \bar{d})^2}{N - 1}} = 4.79$; $s_{\bar{d}}$ = standard

error of the differences $= \dfrac{s_d}{\sqrt{N}} = \dfrac{4.79}{\sqrt{10}} = 1.51$; $t = \dfrac{\bar{d}}{s_{\bar{d}}} = \dfrac{2.6}{1.51} = 1.72$.

mg/dl. The 95% confidence limits set for subsequent daily determinations is $220 \pm 2s$ or 206 to 234 mg/dl. The standard error $= \dfrac{7}{\sqrt{30}} = 1.28$. Hence, subsequent monthly means should be expected to fall within 220 ± 2 SE or approximately 217.4 to 222.6 mg/dl.

Student's t test is used to assess the significance of the difference between two means. For example, we might compare a proposed method for serum glucose against a reference method as shown in Table III. Samples should be selected for this comparison to cover a range of low, normal, and elevated values. Although results are given for only 10 samples, usually 30 or more are used for such comparisons. When experiments are *paired,* as in this example,

$$t = \frac{\bar{d}}{s_{\bar{d}}}$$

where $\bar{d}$ is the difference between the two means and $s_{\bar{d}}$ is the standard error of the mean difference.

In Table III, there were 10 original differences, but these were summed to permit calculation of the mean difference. Thus, one restriction was imposed and 9 degrees of freedom remain. From tables on statistics we find, for 9 degrees of freedom, that t must exceed 2.26 for the difference to be significant at the 5% level ($p = .05$) and must exceed 3.25 to be significant at the 1% level ($p = .01$). Hence, based on the limited data available, we cannot conclude that there is any significant difference in the results by the two methods.

In many experimental situations it is not possible to employ the technique of pairing, e.g., in comparing test results on two different populations. In this case, t is calculated as follows:

$$t = \frac{\bar{x}_1 - \bar{x}_2}{\sqrt{\dfrac{s_1^2}{N_1} + \dfrac{s_2^2}{N_2}}}$$

where $\bar{x}_1$ and $\bar{x}_2$, and s_1 and s_2 are the respective means and standard deviations of the two series of N_1 and N_2 individuals.

In one study, we compared serum albumin concentrations in two groups of males and obtained the following results.

Age group (yrs)	N	Mean albumin (g/dl)	s
70–79	66	3.66	0.40
80–89	56	3.38	0.48

The values were found to be normally distributed in each group. By substitution in the above equation,

$$t = \frac{3.66 - 3.38}{\sqrt{\dfrac{(0.40)^2}{66} + \dfrac{(0.48)^2}{56}}} = 3.46$$

For this nonpaired series there are 120 degrees of freedom. From tables on statistics we find that t must exceed 3.38 for the difference in the means to be significant at the 0.1% level ($p = .001$). Hence we may conclude from this particular study that the difference in serum albumin is highly significant for the two age groups, i.e., the probability is less than 1 in 1000 (p < .001) that this difference could occur by chance alone.

In reporting results of any statistical manipulations we must be very careful to define what we mean. Sometimes a set of values may be reported in the literature, for example, as 120 ± 10, with no explanation as to what "10" represents. The value "± 10" could be interpreted as either one standard deviation, two standard deviations, the standard error, or simply the range of values for the raw data. It is incumbent on all authors reporting data to define specifically the meaning of statistical parameters.

REFERENCES

Allen, E., and Rieman, W., III (1953). *Anal. Chem.* **25**, 1325–1331.

Allen, W. A. (1950). *J. Clin. Endocrinol.* **10**, 71–83.

Amenta, J. A. (1963). *Stand. Methods Clin. Chem.* **4**, 31–38.

Blankenship, J., and Campbell, J. B. (1976). "Laboratory Mathematics. Medical and Biological Applications." Mosby, St. Louis, Missouri.

Bowers, G. N., and McComb, R. B. (1970). *Stand. Methods Clin. Chem.* **6**, 31–40.

Dorwart, W. V., and Chalmers, L. (1975). *Clin. Chem.* **21**, 190–194.

DuBois, D., and DuBois, E. F. (1916). *Arch. Int. Med.* **17**, 863–871.

Fog, J. (1958). *Scand. J. Clin. Lab Invest.* **10**, 246–250, 251–256.

Gaebler, O. H. (1943). *J. Biol. Chem.* **149**, 251–254.

Gaebler, O. H. (1945). *Am. J. Clin. Pathol.* **15**, 452–455.

Goldberg, D. M., Handyside, A. J., and Winfield, D. A. (1973). *Clin. Chem.* **19**, 395–402.

Hidalgo, J. U., Nadler, S. B., and Bloch, T. (1962). *J. Nucl. Med.* **3**, 94–99.

Jatlow, P. (1975). *Clin. Chem.* **21**, 1518–1520.

Kaye, S. (1970). "Handbook of Emergency Toxicology." 3rd ed., Thomas, Springfield, Illinois.

Koch-Weser, J., and Klein, S. W. (1971). *J. Am. Med. Assoc.* **215**, 1454–1460.

Ladenson, J. H., Lewis, J. W., and Boyd, J. C. (1978). *J. Clin. Endocrinol. Metab.* **46**, 986–993.

Levitt, M. D., Johnson, S. G., Ellis, C. J., and Engel, R. R. (1977). *Gastroenterology* **72**, 1260–1263.

McCance, R. A., and Widdowson, E. M. (1952). *Lancet* **2**, 860–862.

McKiel, R. R., and Albertson, D. F. (1978). *Clin. Chem.* **24**, 1016.

McLean, F. C., and Hastings, A. B. (1935). *Am. J. Med. Sci.* **189**, 601–613.

Martin, H. F., Gudzinowicz, B. J., and Fanger, H. (1975). "Normal Values in Clinical Chemistry." Marcel Dekker, New York.

Morgan, D. B., Dillon, S., and Payne, R. B. (1978). *Postgrad. Med. J.* **54**, 302–310.

Nadeau, G. (1954). *Am. J. Clin. Pathol.* **24**, 740–746.

Natelson, S., and Nobel, D. (1977). *Clin. Chem.* **23**, 767–769.

Polanyi, M. L., and Hehir, R. M. (1960). *Rev. Sci. Instrum.* **31**, 401–403.

Reiss, E., and Alexander, F. (1959). *J. Clin. Endocrinol.* **19**, 1212–1222.

Remson, S. T., and Ackermann, P. G. (1977). "Calculations for the Medical Laboratory." Little, Brown, Boston.

Routh, J. I. (1976). "Mathematical Preparation for the Health Sciences." 2nd ed., Saunders, Philadelphia.

Shinowara, G. Y. (1954). *Am. J. Clin. Pathol.* **24**, 696–710.

Shinowara, G. Y., Jones, L. M., and Reinhart, H. L. (1942). *J. Biol. Chem.* **66**, 921–933.

Sunshine, I. (1969). "Handbook of Analytical Toxicology." Chemical Rubber Co., Cleveland.

Warshaw, A. L., and Fuller, A. F. (1975). *N. Engl. J. Med.* **292**, 325–328.

Zeisler, E. B. (1954). *Am. J. Clin. Pathol.* **24**, 588–593.

Blood Gases, pH, and Acid–Base Balance

NORMAN LASKER

I. INTRODUCTION*

Many hospital laboratories routinely perform a blood gas and acid–base profile when ''blood gases'' are ordered. Appropriate electrodes allow the determination of arterial oxygen tension (P_aO_2), arterial carbon dioxide tension (P_aCO_2), and pH on one blood sample. From these, the bicarbonate concentration [HCO_3^-], CO_2 content, base excess, and oxygen

---

* *Glossary:* P_aO_2, oxygen tension in arterial blood; P_aCO_2, carbon dioxide tension in arterial blood; dCO_2, dissolved carbon dioxide; dO_2, dissolved oxygen; Hb^-, deoxygenated

CLINICAL BIOCHEMISTRY
Contemporary Theories and Techniques, Vol. 1

saturation are calculated. A patient in sufficient respiratory distress to warrant an arterial puncture for blood gas determination is likely to benefit from a pH and bicarbonate determination since there is a close association between blood gases and acid–base metabolism. The P_aO_2 and P_aCO_2 can be altered in respiratory and nonrespiratory acid–base disorders. A decrease in ventilation resulting in an increase in a P_aCO_2 will produce respiratory acidosis and compensatory metabolic* alkalosis. An acute increase in pH due to metabolic alkalosis can decrease pulmonary ventilation and the dissociation of oxyhemoglobin with a decrease in tissue oxygenation. Tissue hypoxia can cause the accumulation of lactic acid and produce metabolic acidosis.

To a large extent, tissue oxygenation depends on pulmonary function including ventilation, perfusion and diffusion, the uptake and release of oxygen by hemoglobin as well as cardiac output and regional blood flow. Carbon dioxide's effect on acid–base parameters depends on tissue and renal buffering, CO_2 transport, and pulmonary ventilation.

These topics will be discussed from the viewpoint of respiratory and renal physiology in the earlier sections and from a clinical acid–base orientation in section VI.

II. RESPIRATORY PHYSIOLOGY (9,15)

A. Oxygen

1. Oxygen Saturation

Most of the oxygen carried in the blood is combined with hemoglobin with a relatively small amount present in the aqueous phase as dissolved oxygen. The amount combined with hemoglobin is expressed by the oxygen saturation of hemoglobin, which is the quantity of oxygen bound to the available hemoglobin compared with the quantity that could be bound, designated as a percentage. One gram of fully oxygenated hemo-

---

hemoglobin or reduced hemoglobin; Hb, hemoglobin; HbO_2, oxyhemoglobin: $[H^+]$, hydrogen ion concentration: pH, negative log of hydrogen ion concentration: pK, negative log of dissociation constant: $P(A - a)O_2$, alveolar–arterial oxygen gradient; P_AO_2, oxygen tension in alveolar air; P_ACO_2, carbon dioxide tension in alveolar air; RQ, respiratory quotient; 2,3-DPG, 2,3-diphosphoglycerate; Torr, unit of pressure required to support 1 mm column of mercury at 0°C against acceleration of gravity at 45° N latitude (used in preference to mm Hg); V/Q, ventilation–perfusion ratio.

* Metabolic refers to nonrespiratory acid–base derangements. This term is used although the disorders are not always metabolic in origin, i.e., metabolic acidosis 2° to diarrheal loss of HCO_3 .

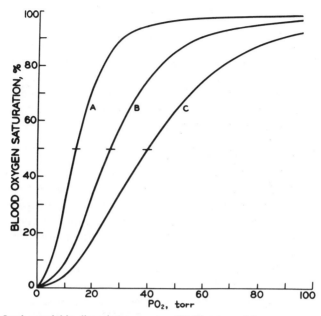

Fig. 1 Oxyhemoglobin dissociation curves. (B) The normal human curve with P50 of 27 mm Hg. (A) and (C) Blood with increased and decreased affinity for oxygen respectively. Reproduced by permission of American Thoracic Society.

globin can carry 1.34 ml of oxygen whereas at an arterial oxygen tension (P_aO_2) of 100 mm Hg the dissolved oxygen is only 0.3 ml/100 ml of blood.

Oxygen saturation can be determined by the Van Slyke manometric technique in which the actual oxygen content of a blood sample is compared with an aliquot that has been fully saturated with oxygen *in vitro*(32). The ratio is calculated after subtracting the dissolved oxygen. The Van Slyke method is very accurate, but more time consuming than spectrophotometric or colorimetric techniques in which the oxygen saturation is determined by the amount of light that is respectively reflected or transmitted by the sample. Oxygen saturation can also be determined by relating the arterial oxygen tension (P_aO_2) to the oxygen saturation on an oxyhemoglobin dissociation curve (Fig. 1). A commonly used method adjusts the oxyhemoglobin curve for pH, which is only one of several determinants of the oxyhemoglobin dissociation curve, e.g., temperature, 2,3-diphosphoglycerate (2,3-DPG), and pCO_2. Therefore, the value obtained by this method may be inaccurate.

The oxyhemoglobin dissociation curve shows the relationship between the blood's oxygen saturation and the P_aO_2. It is a sigmoid-shaped curve (Fig. 1) indicating that at a P_aO_2 over 70 mm Hg the blood is almost fully saturated whereas below a P_aO_2 of 60 mm Hg the oxygen saturation falls off rapidly. Therefore, the blood is highly saturated in the lungs as long as pulmonary capillary P_aO_2 is 70 mm Hg or greater, but at 60 mm Hg or less, insufficient hemoglobin is saturated to provide adequate oxygen delivery to the tissues. The curve also indicates that at the low P_aO_2 of the blood in the peripheral tissues the hemoglobin gives off its oxygen very readily with little drop in P_aO_2. Thus, a favorable pressure gradient for oxygen diffusion into cells is maintained.

2. Arterial Oxygen Tension (P_aO_2)

The arterial oxygen tension (P_aO_2) is in equilibrium with the dissolved oxygen in the blood. Both of these are dependent on several variables including the oxygen concentration and pressure of the inspired and alveolar air, the degree of alveolar–capillary block, the match-up between the alveolar ventilation and perfusion, and the degree of venous–arterial shunting.

The P_aO_2 is usually measured by the Clark electrode, which consists of a platinum anode surrounded by an oxygen-permeable membrane containing an electrolyte solution with an ionic content that is sensitive to oxygen. Current flows between the anode and a silver cathode in proportion to the oxygen-determined ionic content of the electrolyte solution (18).

The magnitude of the alveolar–capillary block or the pulmonary diffusing capacity can be approximated by measuring the difference between the alveolar oxygen tension (P_AO_2) and the P_aO_2 ("alveolar–arterial O_2 gradient"). This gradient can also help to distinguish the elevated pCO_2 due to hypoventilation as in metabolic alkalosis from that due to intrinsic lung disease. (In the former, an increased alveolar–arterial oxygen gradient should not be present.) Measurement of the alveolar–arterial oxygen gradient [$P(A - a)O_2$] first requires the determination of the PAO_2. When breathing room air at sea level PAO_2 is determined as:

$$\frac{P_AO_2}{mm\ Hg} = (760\ mm\ Hg - 47\ mm\ Hg)\ 21\% - \frac{40\ mm\ Hg}{0.8} \tag{1}$$

where 760 mm Hg is the barometric pressure, 47 mm Hg is the water vapor pressure, 21% is the fractional content of oxygen in inspired air,* 40 mm Hg is the P_aCO_2, 0.8 is the respiratory quotient. P_AO_2 is 100 mm Hg.

If P_aO_2 = 90 mm Hg the A − a oxygen gradient is 10 mm Hg (20 mm Hg or less is normal).

The $P(A - a)O_2$ is increased by direct diffusion defects, but more com-

---

* The patient on a respirator may be breathing air with a different fractional oxygen content. This fraction would be substituted for the 21% utilized in this example.

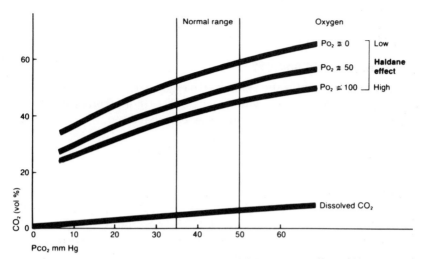

Fig. 2 Relationship between PCO_2, dCO_2, and CO_2 content. Effect of H_b oxygenation on CO_2 buffering. Reprinted with permission of Upjohn Scope Publications.

monly by alveolar O_2 ventilation–perfusion (V/Q) inequality and venous–arterial shunts. In conditions of V/Q inequality some alveoli are either underventilated in relation to perfusion or underperfused in regard to ventilation. In either case, alveolar ventilation is ineffective and pulmonary venous blood will not be adequately oxygenated resulting in a decreased P_aO_2. Examining the oxyhemoglobin dissociation curve (Fig. 1) reveals that increasing the ventilation of the normal alveoli with room air cannot compensate for the abnormal alveoli because the curve is horizontal at its upper ranges indicating that the blood in the normal alveolar capillaries is already fully saturated with oxygen. However, the $PaCO_2$ may be normal or low because the CO_2 dissociation curve is a straight ascending line (Fig. 2) and compensation can occur in the normal alveoli. (CO_2 is also more diffusible than oxygen.) Examples of ventilation–perfusion mismatch include pulmonary embolus, emphysema, obstructive airway disease, atelectasis, and acute respiratory distress syndrome.

Venous arterial shunts allow venous blood to bypass ventilated alveoli so the mixed arterial blood has a lower P_aO_2 than normal. A totally atelectatic or consolidated lung segment that continues to be perfused is an extreme example of ventilation perfusion inequality or, more appropriately, venous–arterial shunting. A patient with diffusion problems or the usual ventilation–perfusion inequality can normalize his P_aO_2 by breathing air with 60–100% oxygen concentration to increase the P_AO_2 in even minimally ventilated alveoli; the individual with significant shunting will remain undersaturated since the P_AO_2 cannot be increased in totally consolidated alveoli and venous blood will continue to mix with the already maximally saturated arterial blood.

3. Oxygen Content and p50

The oxygen content is the amount of oxygen carried by the blood in solution and in combination with hemoglobin. (It is expressed in vol%, which is the same as $cm^3/100 \ cm^3$) It is calculated by:

$$O_2 \ content = \frac{Hb \ conc.}{gm/100 \ cm^3} \times \% \ O_2 \ saturation \times 1.34 \ ml/gm \ Hb$$

$$+ \ 0.003 \ ml \ O_2/100 \ cm^3 \times P_aO_2 \quad (2)$$

Oxygen delivery to the organs depends on three factors: the oxygen content of the blood, the cardiac output, and the position of the oxygen dissociation curve of hemoglobin (Hb). The position of this curve is expressed by the $P50$, which is the P_aO_2 at which the hemoglobin is 50% saturated with oxygen (Fig. 1). An increase in the $P50$ indicates a shift to the right of the dissociation curve resulting in greater oxygen availability to the tissues at any designated hemoglobin concentration or cardiac output. It also indicates that less oxygen is taken up in the lungs at any pulmonary capillary P_aO_2, but this is usually not critical because of the horizontal nature of the upper portion of the oxyhemoglobin dissociation curve with greater than 90% saturation P_aO_2's above 70 mm Hg.

The $P50$ is increased by elevated red blood cell 2,3-DPG, a drop in pH (Bohr effect), an increase in pCO_2, and a rise in temperature. 2,3-DPG is a phosphorylase enzyme in the red blood cell (RBC), which facilitates the release of oxygen from hemoglobin. It is increased by hypoxia, metabolic alkalosis, and hyperphosphatemia; it is decreased in stored blood.

Oxygen delivery to the cells is also dependent on local circulatory factors such as capillary blood flow and the number of capillaries being perfused. When oxygen delivery is inadequate because of systemic or local factors, mitochondrial oxidation is inhibited and anaerobic glycolysis is facilitated. This can result in lactic acidosis (Section VI,C.)

B. Buffer Action and the CO₂ System

By the Bronsted definition an acid is a hydrogen ion (proton) donor and a base is a hydrogen ion acceptor. Carbon dioxide (CO_2) is a potential acid since it can combine with water (H_2O) to form carbonic acid (H_2CO_3). 20,000 mmoles of CO_2 are produced per day by oxidative metabolism of carbohydrate and fats representing a potentially lethal source of acid. It is rendered innocuous by the open system within which it is produced and by the presence of intracellular (particularly hemoglobin) and extracel-

lular buffers. In an open system there is an outlet for a metabolically produced acid or base. The lungs serve this purpose for CO_2 and the kidneys
provide an outlet for strong acids such as H_2SO_4.

1. Buffer Action

A buffer pair is the combination of a weak acid and its conjugate* base
that resists a change in hydrogen ion concentration $[H^+]$. Examples of
conjugate buffer pairs include H_2CO_3 and HCO_3^- and HbO_2 (oxyhemoglobin) and Hb^- (deoxygenated hemoglobin). Proteins can buffer as
Zwitter ions because of the presence of NH_3^+ (amino) groups, which can
act as acids and COO^- (carboxyl) groups which can act as bases.

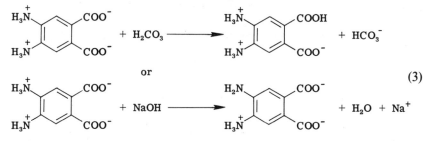

(3)

2. CO₂ Transfer (9)

Carbon dioxide produced in the tissue cells is dissolved in the interstitial fluid and diffuses down a concentration gradient into the plasma (Fig.
3). Most of the CO_2 is present as dCO_2 (dissolved carbon dioxide) and
very little as H_2CO_3 because interstitial fluid and plasma lack carbonic anhydrase that facilitates the reaction between dCO_2 and H_2O to form
H_2CO_3.

$$dCO_2 + H_2O \xleftrightarrow{\text{Carbonic anhydrase}} H_2CO_3 \longleftrightarrow H^+ + HCO_3^- \qquad (4)$$

The ratio of dCO_2 to H_2CO_3 in the plasma is approximately 700 to 1.
H_2CO_3 formed in the plasma is buffered primarily by plasma proteins and
a small amount of dCO_2 is attached to plasma proteins as carbamino compounds:

$$R{-}NH_2 + CO_2 \longleftrightarrow R{-}NHCOO^- + H^+ \text{ (buffered by plasma buffers)} \qquad (5)$$
$$\text{Protein} \qquad\qquad \text{Carbamino}$$
$$\text{compound}$$

The bulk of the CO_2 diffuses into the RBC where it either forms carbamino compounds with hemoglobin or combines with H_2O to form H_2CO_3
due to the large concentration of carbonic anhydrase in the RBC. H_2CO_3

---

* Conjugate base, usually an anion remaining after acid gives off a hydrogen ion.

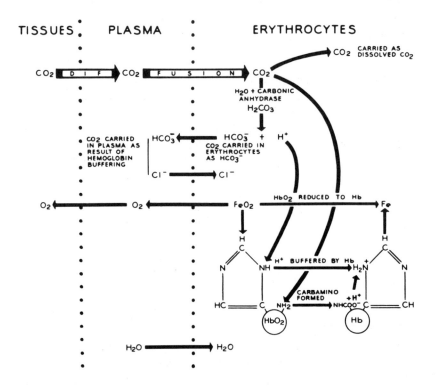

Fig. 3 Schematic representation of the processes occurring when CO_2 passes from tissues into RBCs. From H. W. Davenport (5) with permission.

dissociates into HCO_3^- and H^+ with the H^+ buffered mainly by reduced (deoxygenated) Hb. The HCO_3^- diffuses into the plasma down its concentration gradient and chloride (Cl^-) shifts into the RBC to maintain electroneutrality. 63% of the CO_2 produced in the tissues is carried as plasma HCO_3^-, 29% as carbamino groups (mainly attached to hemoglobin), and 8% as dissolved CO_2 (mainly in the plasma). It is the buffering of H^+ by hemoglobin which allows the bulk of CO_2 to be transported. This buffering is enhanced by the reduced acidity of deoxygenated Hb. This ability of reduced hemoglobin to carry more carbon dioxide is called the Haldane effect.

When the blood reaches the lungs, the dissolved CO_2 in the plasma at a partial pressure of 46 mm Hg equilibrates with the lower CO_2 tension of the alveoli (40 mm Hg) to bring the arterial P_aCO_2 to 40 mm Hg. Reduced hemoglobin is oxygenated and becomes a stronger acid, releasing hydrogen ions. These react with HCO_3^- to form H_2CO_3, which breaks down to CO_2 and H_2O under the influence of carbonic anhydrase in the RBC. Utilization of RBC bicarbonate causes plasma HCO_3^- to shift into the RBC and Cl^- to exit into the plasma. The oxygenated Hb also gives off its carbamino CO_2. The CO_2 accumulated in the RBC enters the plasma as dissolved CO_2 and rapidly diffuses into the alveoli as gaseous CO_2. The alveolar membrane barrier is 20 times more permeable to CO_2 than it is to O_2 and CO_2 equilibration between blood and alveolar air is achieved within 0.01 sec.

3. Evaluation of Ventilation

The central chemoreceptor cells that control ventilation are highly sensitive to changes in local hydrogen ion concentration produced by alterations in dCO_2. Any change in carbon dioxide production has little effect on the plasma dCO_2 (or its associated pCO_2) because an immediate adjustment will increase or decrease ventilation until the carbon dioxide concentration is normal. This chemoreceptor sensitivity and the high permeability of the alveolar barrier to CO_2 makes the plasma P_aCO_2 a valid index of pulmonary ventilation and the usual indicator of respiratory acid–base disturbances.

4. CO_2 Measurement

Blood tension of CO_2 (pCO_2) is measured with a Severinghaus electrode. This consists of a pH electrode surrounded by a HCO_3^- solution within a semipermeable membrane which is permeable to dCO_2 but not to HCO_3^-. Dissolved CO_2 in the blood diffuses into the HCO_3^- solution changing its pH in proportion to the concentration of dCO_2 that is in equilibrium with pCO_2 (28).

III. MEASUREMENT OF THE METABOLIC COMPONENT

A. Plasma Techniques

Just as the plasma pCO_2 is the usual indicator of respiratory acid–base disorders, the plasma $[HCO_3^-]$ is the usual guide in metabolic acid–base disorders. In an anephric animal extracellular HCO_3^- buffers about one-half of an acute fixed* acid load while intracellular buffers take care of the rest (23). The HCO_3^- is converted to H_2CO_3 and expired by the lungs as

---

* Fixed acids are nonvolatile acids such as HCl or H_2SO_4 whereas CO_2 is considered a volatile acid.

CO_2. Two-thirds of an acute alkali load is buffered extracellularly in an anephric animal with a resultant increase in $[HCO_3^-]$ (23).

1. CO₂ Content

The CO_2 content is the sum of the serum or plasma $[HCO_3^-]$, dissolved CO_2, and the plasma carbamino CO_2. Since the dissolved CO_2 and plasma carbamino CO_2 are relatively small moieties, the CO_2 content is practically synonymous with HCO_3^- concentration $[HCO_3^-]$. The test is performed by collecting the venous blood and separating the serum or plasma anaerobically. The serum is acidified converting the HCO_3^- to H_2CO_3, which in turn forms dissolved CO_2. The sample is then exposed to a negative pressure, which causes all the CO_2 plus the other gases to enter the enclosed atmosphere. NaOH is then added to form Na_2CO_3 (carbonate) with the CO_2 removing it from the gas phase. The difference between the original total gas volume and the volume remaining after the addition of NaOH represents the CO_2 content of the sample.

2. CO₂ Combining Power

Since both respiratory and metabolic disturbances alter the bicarbonate concentration (see Section V,A) there have been several attempts to adapt the bicarbonate measurement to more truly reflect a primary "metabolic" disorder. (These approaches were more prevalent when pH determinations were not readily available.) The CO_2 combining power was one of these attempts to negate the respiratory influence on $[HCO_3^-]$. It is based on the concept that if the plasma is returned to a normal pCO_2 of 40 mm Hg the respiratory influence on $[HCO_3^-]$ will be negated. Venous blood is not usually collected under anaerobic conditions. The separated plasma is equilibrated with 5.5% carbon dioxide (40 mm Hg PCO_2) at room temperature. The sample is acidified to convert the HCO_3^- to H_2CO_3, negative pressure is applied, and the extracted CO_2 is measured. At a pCO_2 of 40 mm Hg the dissolved CO_2 is 1.2 mmoles/liter and this is subtracted from the total. Since the CO_2 equilibration is performed with plasma the amount of buffering is less than that available in whole blood because of the lack of hemoglobin. If the blood sample loses CO_2 to a level below 40 mm Hg before the plasma is separated, the equilibrated plasma will have a lower $[HCO_3^-]$ than equilibrated whole blood; on the other hand, if the blood has a high $[HCO_3^-]$ and pCO_2, equilibration as plasma with 40 mm Hg pCO_2 would give a falsely high $[HCO_3^-]$ because of decreased buffering. Performing the equilibration at room temperature instead of 38°C is another source of error.

Both the CO_2 content and CO_2 combining power can be determined with automated systems. The plasma or serum is aspirated and segmented with CO_2-free air. It is then acidified and the liberated CO_2 is allowed to segment an alkaline buffer stream containing a pH indicator. The change in color is read spectrophotometrically in a flow through curvette. Standards are run in between samples for quantitation. The CO_2 combining power is performed following the equilibration of the plasma with 5.5% CO_2.

B. Whole Blood Techniques

1. Standard Bicarbonate

Standard bicarbonate compensates for many of the inadequacies of the CO_2 combining power by equilibrating whole blood *in vitro* with a gas mixture of CO_2 and oxygen at 38°C. The pCO_2 of the mixture is 40 mm Hg. The fully oxygenated blood is separated and all the CO_2 in the plasma is extracted and measured as described for CO_2 combining power. The standard bicarbonate can be obtained by measuring the pH of the plasma from fully equilibrated blood and substituting in the Henderson–Hasselbalch equation with a pCO_2 of 40 mm Hg [see Eq. (7), Section V,A]. It can also be derived from the oxygenated bloods log pCO_2 − pH buffer line utilizing the Siggaard Andersen nomogram (Fig. 4) (29).

The deviation of the standard bicarbonate from normal has been used to quantitate the fixed acid or base accumulation, but since it utilizes an *in vitro* CO_2 titration curve, it may not accurately reflect the *in vivo* curve where extravascular CO_2 buffering can occur and where HCO_3^- formed by Hb^- buffering of CO_2 can move interstitially.

2. Whole Blood Buffer Base (WBB) and Base Excess

The whole blood buffer base (WBB) has been used to quantitate the gain or loss of fixed acid or base. It is the sum of the concentration of all buffer anions in the whole blood including bicarbonate, hemoglobin, plasma proteins, and phosphate (nearly all is due to $[HCO_3^-]$ and Hb^-). It can be measured by titrating whole blood with a strong acid until no further decrease in pH occurs or by using a Singer Hastings nomogram in which two of the three classical plasma acid–base parameters (pH, pCO_2, or $[HCO_3^-]$) and Hb or hematocrit are plotted (30). The deviation of the WBB from normal is thought to reflect the amount of fixed acid or base accumulation. Since the addition of CO_2 to whole blood will increase $[HCO_3^-]$ to the same extent it reduces the non-HCO_3^- buffer concentration respiratory changes should not effect WBB:

$$CO_2 + H_2O \longrightarrow H_2CO_3$$

$$H_2CO_3 + Hb^- \longrightarrow HHb + NaHCO_3$$

(6)

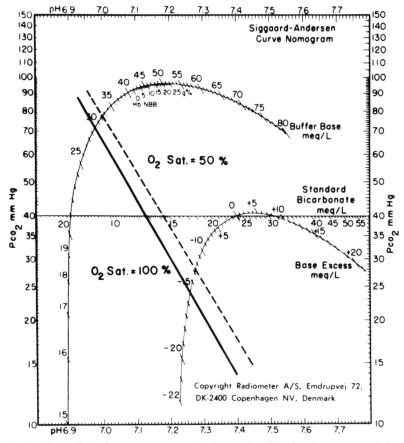

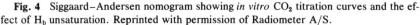

Fig. 4 Siggaard–Andersen nomogram showing *in vitro* CO_2 titration curves and the effect of H_b unsaturation. Reprinted with permission of Radiometer A/S.

The base excess, a concept popularized by Astrup (4) is the difference between the normal buffer base corrected for the blood hemoglobin concentration and the existing blood buffer base. Unlike the Singer Hastings WBB it is measured with fully oxygenated Hb and is, therefore, not influenced by the oxygen saturation of the blood. It is usually obtained by the Astrup technique utilizing a log pCO_2 − pH buffer line superimposed on the Siggaard Andersen nomogram (Fig. 4). The patient's heparinized whole blood is equilibrated with a low and high pCO_2–oxygen mixture to give two pH readings. These are plotted on the nomogram to give the buffer line. The point where the line crosses the pCO_2 40 mm Hg line is the standard bicarbonate and its crossing of the buffer base and base excess curves gives their values. Plotting the pH of the orginal nonequilibrated blood sample on the buffer line allows the pCO_2 to be read directly from the ordinate.

The defect in the standard bicarbonate, WBB and base excess concepts is their dependence on an *in vitro* log CO_2 − pH buffer line. *In vivo* buffering includes non-RBC intracellular buffers as well as bone buffering. HCO_3^- formed during *in vivo* buffering can distribute into a large interstitial volume, which will change the plasma concentration. A fall in intravascular HCO_3^- concentration may be partially corrected by the diffusion of interstitial HCO_3^-. Since these factors are not predictable in an individual patient, there is no reason to expect the *in vitro* blood buffer line to be the same as the *in vivo* whole body buffer line (25).*

The use of the base excess measurement to calculate base or acid therapy assumes that the variation of base excess from normal reflects a pathological process. But changes in WBB or base excess can be due to normal secondary renal adjustments of $[HCO_3^-]$ in response to chronic changes in pCO_2. They do not require correction unless they are inappropriate. Therefore, it is preferable to use the pH, pCO_2, and $[HCO_3^-]$ or CO_2 content in evaluating acid–base problems. An accurate measurement of these perameters combined with a good history and physical and knowledge of the appropriate secondary response to primary acid–base disorders (Table II) is a better guide to therapy than base excess or buffer base alone.

The development of a reliable CO_2 electrode has decreased the use of the Astrup technique since one of the chief advantages of the latter was the ease of obtaining a P_aCO_2 value as compared with the time-consuming manometric technique.

IV. RENAL PHYSIOLOGY

A. Introduction

The kidney's role in normal acid–base metabolism is twofold. It reabsorbs the HCO_3^- that is filtered at the glomerulus and produces new HCO_3^- to replace body losses due to the buffering of fixed acid. The former function is performed mainly by the proximal tubule whereas the latter is performed by the distal convoluted tubule and collecting tubule. There is

---

* In acute respiratory alkalosis, the *in vitro* blood buffer line is the same as the *in vivo* line. This may be due to the balancing of the *in vivo* intravascular movement of HCO_3^- by the *in vivo* production of lactic acid (33).

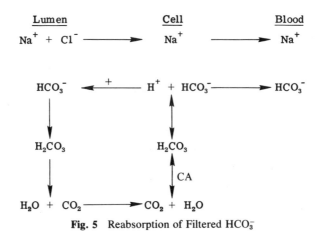

Fig. 5 Reabsorption of Filtered HCO_3^-

approximately 1 mmole/kg of fixed acid produced per day chiefly as H_2SO_4 from protein metabolism and H_3PO_4 from phospholipid metabolism with a small amount of lactic and other organic acids. In the process of buffering this acid, HCO_3^- is converted to H_2CO_3, which is expired by the lungs as CO_2.

B. HCO_3^- Reabsorption (See Fig. 5)

Both the reabsorption of filtered HCO_3^- and the production of new HCO_3^- requires the tubular secretion of H^+. The H^+ comes from H_2CO_3 whose formation in the tubular cell is catalyzed by carbonic anhydrase. The secretion of H^+ by the tubular cells is an active process but it is linked to Na^+ reabsorption by the tubular cells. It is also related to chloride (Cl^-) reabsorption, e.g., in respiratory acidosis as H^+ secretion is enhanced the preferential H^+–Na^+ exchange results in Cl^- loss.

In the proximal tubule the breakdown of luminal H_2CO_3 to CO_2 and H_2O is enhanced by carbonic anhydrase present on the luminal surface.

C. New HCO_3^- Formation

1. Titratable Acid (See Fig. 6)

The distal nephron produces new HCO_3^- by the formation of titratable acid and ammonia (NH_3), which allows adequate distal H^+ secretion to occur. Most of the HCO_3^- has been reabsorbed proximally and the concentration of free hydrogen ions at the lowest urine pH of ~ 4.4 does not allow sufficient H^+ secretion to produce the needed bicarbonate. Titratable acid is defined as the number of milliequivalents of NaOH required to titrate

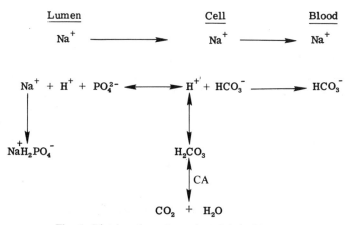

Fig. 6 Distal nephron formation of titratable acid.

the urine back to the pH of the blood. It consists mainly of sodium and potassium dihydrogen phosphate (NaH_2PO_4) and a small amount of other weak acids such as creatinine. Titratable acid is a limited source of HCO_3^- formation because of the finite amount of phosphate that can be filtered.

2. NH₃ Formation (See Fig. 7)

In contrast to the limited formation of titratable acid, NH_3 formation can be greatly augmented. The normal ammonium excretion of 30–50

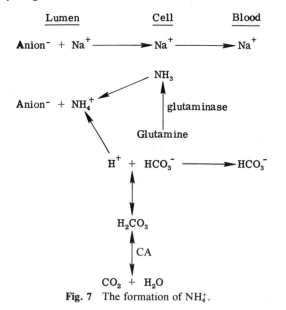

Fig. 7 The formation of NH_4^+.

mEq/day can be increased as much as 10-fold in response to chronic acidosis.

NH$_3$ is formed in the tubular cell by the action of glutaminase on amino acids such as glutamine. Its production is stimulated both by acidosis and hypokalemia. NH$_3$ is freely diffusible through the tubular cell membrane and can passively diffuse down its concentration gradient into the tubular lumen. In the lumen it reacts with H$^+$ to form ammonium (NH$_4^+$), which, unlike NH$_3$, is not readily diffusible. Since the passive NH$_3$ secretion depends on its diffusion gradient, the secretion of H$^+$ and its combination with NH$_3$ to form NH$_4^+$ increases the gradient and allows more NH$_3$ to diffuse into the lumen.

V. MEASUREMENT OF pH AND ACID–BASE STATUS

A. Measurement of pH

pH is the negative log of the [H$^+$] (pH = $-$log [H$^+$]). It is measured with a potentiometer, which measures the electrical potential between two solutions, one having a known standard hydrogen ion activity and the other having the unknown hydrogen ion activity. A glass bulb acting as a semipermeable membrane only permeable to hydrogen ions is filled with a standard buffered solution. A wire passes from the standard solution to one terminal of the potentiometer while the circuit is completed by connecting the unknown solution through a saturated KCl salt bridge to a calomel electrode attached to the other terminal of the potentiometer. The potential difference between the standard and unknown solution is proportional to the hydrogen ion activity. The hydrogen ion activity of the standard solution is constant so the pH meter reads the hydrogen ion activity of the unknown. Most physiological solutions have a very low [H$^+$] and the hydrogen ion activity is practically the same as the [H$^+$]. This is not true of gastric juices where the high [H$^+$] can significantly decrease the hydrogen ion activity and the pH meter may read 25% below the true hydrogen ion concentration (9).

The pH of the plasma is determined by the relationship between pCO$_2$ and [HCO$_3^-$] as defined by the Henderson–Hasselbalch equation:

$$\text{pH} = \text{p}K + \log \frac{\text{base}}{\text{acid}}$$

$$\text{pH} = 6.1 + \log \frac{\text{HCO}_3^-}{d\text{CO}_2 + \text{H}_2\text{CO}_3} \tag{7}$$

$$\text{pH} = 6.1 + \log \frac{\text{HCO}_3^-}{p\text{CO}_2 \times 0.03} = 6.1 + \log \frac{24 \text{ mmoles/liter}}{1.2 \text{ mmoles/liter}}$$

pK is the negative log of the dissociation constant of an acid. The higher the pK the weaker the acid and vice versa. The pK of 6.1 is appropriate to the conditions in the plasma where most of the CO_2 is present as dissolved CO_2 and not H_2CO_3. H_2CO_3 is a relatively strong acid and has a lower pK.

Since the pK is equal to that pH where the buffering effect is greatest the pK of an ideal plasma buffer should be 7.4. The CO_2–HCO_3^- system compensates for this apparent inadequacy by its unique acid component whose concentration can be maintained by the lungs.

The Henderson–Hasselbalch equation can be used to determine any one of the three unknowns when the other two are known. In the usual blood gas determination the pO_2, pCO_2, and pH are determined with electrodes and the bicarbonate is derived from a graph based on the Henderson–Hasselbalch equation. The simpler Henderson equation has greater bedside applicability because it requires no calculation of dissolved CO_2 from pCO_2 and no logarithims. The Henderson equation can be expressed as (17):

$$[H^+] = \frac{24 \times pCO_2 \text{ (mm Hg)}}{HCO_3^- \text{ or } CO_2 \text{ content (mmoles/liter)}} \tag{8}$$

Fortunately, there is almost a linear inverse relationship between $[H^+]$ and pH when $[H^+]$ is expressed in nanoequivalents/liter (16). This is shown in Table I.

TABLE I

Relationship between pH and
Hydrogen Ion Concentration $[H^+]$

pH	$[H+]$	
7.60	20	$(25)^a$
7.50	30	(32)
7.40	40	(40)
7.30	50	(50)
7.20	60	(63)

[a] The actual values for hydrogen ion concentration are shown in parentheses, but for most clinical purposes the 10 progression is adequate. If a more accurate determination of [H] is desired, the normal $[H+]$ of 40 mEq/liter should be multiplied by 1.25 for each 0.1 decrease in pH from 7.4 and multiplied by 0.8 for each 0.1 increase in pH above 7.4 (10).

Based on this inverse progression the $[H^+]$ can be obtained from the pH by substracting the pH fraction from 80, i.e., at a pH of 7.30 the $[H^+]$ is $80-30 = 50$ mEq/liter. It now becomes a simple task to check on the mathematical validity of a set of acid base values by substituting them into the Henderson equation [Eq. (8)]. If the $[HCO_3^-]$ derived from the "blood gas" pCO_2 and pH determination does not check with the CO_2 content obtained by direct measurement, a new pCO_2, or pH, value can be obtained by substituting the CO_2 content value into the Henderson equation. Clinical judgement should indicate which two of the three measured values, i.e., pH, pCO_2, or CO_2 content is correct.

Example: Patient is known to have chronic metabolic acidosis

Laboratory results: pH = 7.58, pCO_2 = 30 mm Hg,

$$[HCO_3^-] = 30 \text{ mmoles/liter (calculated from}$$

$$\text{blood gas analysis)}$$

$$CO_2 \text{ content} = 16 \text{ mmoles/liter}$$

$$\text{(measured by chemistry laboratory)}$$

Blood gas values will check since the $[HCO_3^-]$ is calculated from the pH and pCO_2 (unless the technician read the HCO_3^- incorrectly from the table). However, substituting the measured CO_2 content into the Henderson equation, and solving for pH gives:

$$[H^+] = \frac{24 \times 30}{16} \text{ and } [H^+] = 45 \text{ nEq/liter}$$

Therefore, the pH = 7.35. This is more appropriate to the clinical situation and suggests the original pH measurement and the derived $[HCO_3^-]$ were incorrect.

B. Acid–Base Status

The classification of acid–base disorders is simplified by knowing the normal compensatory response to a primary disturbance. Several studies have been compiled to produce Table II (2, 3, 6, 7, 11, 14).

The primary disturbance is designated as one and the secondary change as some fraction or multiple of one. Knowing these normal values can help determine if a patients response is appropriate, whether a simple or mixed disturbance is present, and the type of therapy indicated.

A normal secondary response to a *simple* acid–base disturbance *will not* completely correct the primary change in pH. However, if one considers the normal range of blood pH as 7.36–7.44 the change in pH may not

TABLE II

Normal Compensatory Response to Simple
Acid–Base Disturbances

Condition	[HCO$_3^-$] (mmole/liter)	CO$_2$ (mm Hg)
Metabolic acidosis	↓ 1	↓ 1.2
Metabolic alkalosis	↑ 1	↑ 0.6
Chronic respiratory alkalosis	↓ .5	↓ 1
Chronic respiratory acidosis	↑ .4	↑ 1
Acute respiratory alkalosis	↓ .2	↓ 1
Acute respiratory acidosis	↑ .1	↑ 1

be appreciated. Particularly in chronic respiratory alkalosis, the renal response is so efficient that the pH may be in the normal range (20).

VI. CLINICAL DISTURBANCES OF ACID–BASE METABOLISM (9, 16, 21)

A. Respiratory Acidosis

Respiratory acidosis results from an accumulation of CO_2 due to inadequate ventilation. The accumulation of H^+ resulting from the formation of H_2CO_3 is inhibited by two buffer reactions, which produce HCO_3^-. Buffering by intracellular buffers such as hemoglobin, phosphate, and proteins is the first reaction. HCO_3^- cannot buffer H_2CO_3 since each H^+ buffered by HCO_3^- would form a new molecule of H_2CO_3. (A small amount of CO_2 buffering by protein occurs extracellularly.) These processes can be shown as:

$$Na^+Buf^- + H_2CO_3 \longleftrightarrow H^+Buf^- + NaHCO_3^- \qquad (9)$$

The intracellular buffering process in peripheral tissues causes the addition of Na^+ and K^+ to the extracellular fluid in exchange for H^+ while Cl^- is shifted into the RBC and HCO_3^- diffuses extracellularly (Fig. 3).

The other mechanism that inhibits the accumulation of free hydrogen ions is an increased renal production of HCO_3^-. As shown by the Henderson reaction, an increase in the [HCO_3^-] will decrease the rise in [H^+] due to CO_2 accumulation [see Eq. (8)].

The intracellular buffering reaction begins almost immediately after pCO_2 is increased but it has a limited effect resulting in a maximum rise of $[HCO_3^-]$ of 3–4 mmoles/liter (Table II). Renal correction begins several hours after a decrease in ventilation and reaches a maximum in 3–4 days. It has a greater capacity than the intracellar buffer mechanism and mainly involves the increased production of H^+ by the carbonic anhydrase system and NH_3^- by the glutaminase system (see Section IV) The former prevents the urinary loss of the filtered HCO_3^- and the latter provides intraluminal H^+ buffering so that new HCO^- can be added to the blood. The preferential facilitation of tubular H^+–Na^+ exchange results in less Na^+ absorption with Cl^-. More Cl^- is lost in association with NH_4^+ as $NH_4^+Cl^-$.

The causes of respiratory acidosis can be divided into acute or chronic. The acute causes usually last for a few hours and are relatively poorly buffered whereas the chronic causes persist long enough for full renal compensation. (See Table III and IV)

The result of the renal adaption to chronic respiratory acidosis is an increase in blood $[HCO_3^-]$ and a decreased blood $[Cl^-]$. When a steady state of acidosis or hypercapnia (increased pCO_2 in blood) is reached, the excretion of CO_2 equals the production because the high blood–alveolar CO_2 gradient overcomes the effect of decreased pulmonary ventilation.

TABLE III

Causes of Acute Respiratory Acidosis

Neuromuscular
   Cerebral trauma or infarction
   High cord injury
   Guillain Barre syndrome
   Botulism
   Myasthenia gravis
   Drugs—sedatives/analgesics, curare, aminoglycosides
Airway obstruction
   Aspiration of foreign body or vomitus
   Laryngospasm
   Severe bronchospasm
Thoracic—pulmonary disorders
   Flail chest
   Pneumothorax
   Severe pneumonitis
   Smoke inhalation
   Severe pulmonary edema
Vascular disease
   Massive pulmonary embolism

TABLE IV

Causes of Chronic Respiratory Acidosis

Neuromuscular abnormalities
    Chronic narcotic or sedative ingestion
    Primary hypoventilation
    Pickwickian syndrome
    Poliomyelitis
    Muscle paralysis
Thoracic–pulmonary disorders
    Chronic obstructive lung disease
    Kyphoscoliosis
    End-stage interstitial pulmonary disease

The treatment of acute respiratory acidosis is urgent because of the comparatively large fall in pH and the hypoxia associated with hypoventilation. The primary consideration is establishment of an airway and artificial ventilation as indicated. Antagonists such as Narcan for opiates and Neostigmine for curare overdosage may provide temporary improvement as well as diagnostic information. Severe acidosis tends to increase catecholamine release and has a direct vasodilating effect on the peripheral arterioles and a vasoconstricting effect on the venules. Coupled with a direct depressant effect on the myocardium these actions can result in a markedly unstable cardiac output and blood pressure (8). It may occasionally be necessary to treat the acidosis with intravenous HCO_3^- but the optimum therapy is reestablishment of adequate ventilation.

Chronic respiratory acidosis is tolerated much better than the acute variety. Treatment consists of "correcting the correctible" such as acute pneumonitis or bronchitis superimposed on chronic pulmonary conditions. Chronic exposure to a high concentration of carbon dioxide can depress the cerebral respiratory centers and the hypoxic drive to the peripheral chemoreceptors may become the main stimulus to respiration. The provision of a high concentration of oxygen by nasal catheter or mask may remove this hypoxic stimulus and result in a dangerous depression of respiration.

During the renal adjustment to chronic respiratory acidosis, Cl^- is lost in the urine. Since these patients are frequently on diuretics and salt-restricted diets because of congestive heart failure the Cl^- deficit is magnified. The correction of the CO_2 retention by medical or mechanical means may leave the patient with an elevated HCO_3^- and metabolic alkalosis, which requires the replacement of Cl^- for correction (see Section VI,C)

B. Respiratory Alkalosis

Respiratory alkalosis results from a decrease in pCO_2 due to hyperventilation. The loss of CO_2 will tend to lower the $[H^+]$ [see Eq. (8)].

The same intracellular buffer pairs involved in buffering acute respiratory acidosis by absorbing H^+ will now provide H^+ to lower the blood $[HCO_3^-]$ and minimize the change in $[H^+]$:

$$H^+Buf^- + NaHCO_3 \longleftrightarrow Na^+Buf^- + H_2CO_3$$
$$\updownarrow$$
$$CO_2 + H_2O \qquad\qquad (10)$$

The maximum fall in $[HCO_3^-]$ in acute respiratory alkalosis is 3–4 mmoles/liter (see Table II). After 3–4 h of respiratory alkalosis, the kidneys respond by excreting HCO_3^- with a maximum response in about 3 days.

The cause of the increased renal loss and decreased production of HCO_3^- is a decrease in the carbonic anhydrase mediated production of H^+ by the renal tubular cells in response to the low CO_2 and decreased production of NH_3 resulting from the alkalosis. The former allows filtered HCO_3^- to be excreted as Na^+ and $K^+HCO_3^-$ whereas the latter decreases the production of new HCO_3^- to replace that lost in buffering the normal daily load of fixed acid.

Since the causes of acute respiratory alkalosis may persist to result in chronic respiratory alkalosis, they are not listed separately. (See Table V)

The "peripheral" causes of respiratory stimulation are usually associated with hypoxemia or decreased P_aO_2. Early in alkalosis there is also a shift of the oxyhemoglobin dissociation curve to the left while the decrease in pCO_2 can cause vasoconstriction particularly in the cerebral circulation. These factors can combine to produce dangerous tissue hy-

TABLE V

Causes of Respiratory Alkalosis

Central stimulation of respiration	Uncertain etiology
Anxiety and hysteria	Hepatic insufficiency
Head trauma	Gram-negative septicemia
Vascular accidents or brain tumors	Mechanical hyperventilation
Salicylates	
Fever	
Peripheral stimulation of respiration	
Pulmonary emboli	
Congestive heart failure	
Interstitial lung disease	
Pneumonia	
High altitudes	

poxia. Patients on mechanical ventilators may benefit from increasing the dead space or adding 3% CO_2 for short periods, but the primary consideration is correcting hypoxia and the underlying etiology.

Alkalosis may lower the serum K^+ by promoting the movement of K^+ and Na^+ into tissue cells in exchange for H^+. Hypokalemia coupled with the effects of hypoxia, previous digitalization, or cardiac disease can lead to serious arrythmias.

Another clinical manifestation of respiratory alkalosis is increased neuromuscular irritability ascribed to a decrease ionized calcium. This may present with paresthesias, hyperreflexia, tetany and seizures (24). It may temporarily respond to rebreathing into a paper bag while the underlying cause of hyperventialation is corrected.

C. Metabolic Acidosis

Metabolic acidosis results from a gain of fixed acid or loss of base $[HCO_3^-]$ from the body. It is characterized by a decrease in $[HCO_3^-]$ and a tendency to increase $[H^+]$ in the blood. The decrease in $[HCO_3^-]$ is due to GI or renal losses, the dilution of plasma $[HCO_3^-]$ or buffering of an acid load.

There are three buffer mechanisms that attempt to minimize the rise in $[H^+]$. The first is tissue buffering, which is mainly intracellular, involving such buffers as Hb, protein, and phosphate. Over 50% of an acute acid load is buffered intracellularly. The second is an increase in respiration due to the stimulation of the medullary respiratory center by the increase in $[H^+]$. Although the pCO_2 may not reach its lowest level for 12–24 h, most of the response is so rapid and predictable that it allows for a simple HCO_3^-–pCO_2 relationship with a range of 1 to 1.0–1.5 (Table II). The third buffer mechanism is renal and depends primarily on an increase in the production of NH_3 due to H^+ stimulation of the glutaminase system. This results in an increased production of HCO_3^- (Fig. 7), which reaches a maximum in 4–5 days. The fall in pCO_2 associated with metabolic acidosis decreases the activity of the tubular carbonic anhydrase system, but since less HCO_3^- is filtered tubular H^+ secretion is usually adequate to absorb the decreased amount of filtered HCO_3^- and produce an acid urine.

Metabolic acidosis can be divided into two types based on the anion gap. The first is associated with an increase in the anion gap whereas the anion gap is normal in the second but the $[Cl^-]$ is increased. Actually the anion gap is an artifact resulting from the manner of reporting electrolyte results. Electroneutrality requires that the anions balance the cations in body fluids, but the only anions reported in an electrolyte screen are Cl^- and HCO_3^-. The unreported anions include albumin, sulfate, phosphate, and anions of organic acids. If the sum of $[Cl^-]$ and $[HCO_3^-]$ is subtracted from $[Na^+]$ the difference is normally 10–14 mEq/liter, representing the normal anion gap.

$$[Na^+] = 140 \text{ mEq/liter} \qquad 140-128 = 12 \text{ mEq/liter (normal anion gap)}$$
$$[Cl^-] = 104 \text{ mEq/liter}$$
$$[HCO^-] = 24 \text{ mEq/liter}$$

When a fixed acid such as acetoacetic acid is added to the body fluids it is first buffered by plasma HCO_3^- resulting in:

$$NaHCO_3 + \text{acetoacetic acid} \longrightarrow H_2CO_3 + Na \text{ acetoacetate} \qquad (11)$$

If Na acetoacetate is not excreted or metabolized to form new HCO_3^- the result is a fall in HCO_3^- and a rise in the anion gap.

Metabolic acidosis without an increase in anion gap is associated with the replacement of HCO_3^- by Cl^-. An example would be the addition of HCl to the blood:

$$NaHCO_3 + HCl \longrightarrow NaCl + H_2CO_3 \qquad (12)$$

Table VI lists causes of metabolic acidosis.

Ketoacidosis is due to an accumulation of B-OH butyric acid and acetoacetic acid in conditions such as diabetic ketoacidosis, alcholic ketoacidosis, and starvation ketoacidosis where increased amounts of fat are catabolized.

Lactic acidosis usually results from tissue hypoxia, which causes an increase in anaerobic glycolysis and a decrease in hepatic uptake of lactate. Normally lactic acid, which is the end product of anaerobic glycolysis, is in equilibrium with pyruvic acid. The ratio of lactate to pyruvate depends

TABLE VI

Causes of Metabolic Acidosis

Increased anion gap	Normal anion gap—hyperchloremic
Increased acid production	Increased GI losses of HCO_3^-
Ketoacidosis	Diarrhea
Lactic acidosis	Small bowel, pancreatic, or biliary drainage
Ingestion of toxic substances	Ureterosigmoidostomy or obstructed ileal loop
Ethylene glycol ingestion	Anion exchange resins (Cholestyramine)
Methyl alcohol ingestion	Renal loss of HCO_3^-
Paraldehyde overdose	Carbonic anhydrase inhibitors RTA
Salicylate overdose	Miscellaneous
Failure to excrete fixed acids	Hyperalimentation
Renal failure	Dilutional
	Addition of HCl or NH_4Cl

on the ratio between nicatinamide adenine dinucleotide (NAD) and NADH. NADH promotes the conversion of pyrurate to lactate and NAD promotes the conversion of lactate to pyruvate. Pyruvate can be converted to CO_2 and H_2O through the tricarboxylic acid cycle but lactate can only be converted back to pyruvate. This conversion reaction also requires lactic dehydrogrenase (LDH):

$$\text{Pyruvate} \underset{\underset{\text{LDH}}{\longleftarrow}}{\overset{\text{NADH}}{\underset{\text{NAD}}{\longrightarrow}}} \text{Lactate} \tag{13}$$

NADH is converted to NAD by oxidation in the mitochondria and this conversion is inhibited by hypoxia causing further lactic acid accumulation.

The normal ratio of lactate to pyruvate is 10 to 1 with a lactate concentration of 0.3–1.3 mmoles/liter. In some relatively benign conditions both lactate and pyruvate are increased due to an increase in glycolysis. This may be seen with respiratory alkalosis, hyperalimentation, and increased sympathetic activity. In more serious states associated with tissue hypoxia including hypoxemia ($P_aO_2 < 35$ mm Hg) shock, severe anemia, and drugs, such as Phenformin, lactic acid accumulation is accelerated and the lactate–pyruvate ratio is increased.

In both keotacidosis and lactic acidosis the accumulated anions represent potential sources of base if they are metabolized. This must be considered when estimating the therapeutic bicarbonate requirement during the early recovery phase.

The ingestion of paraldehyde, methyl alcohol, and ethylene glycol can lead to the accumulation of organic acids and high anion gap metabolic acidosis. The responsible metabolite in paraldehyde acidosis is not known. Methyl alcohol is metabolized to formic acid, which inhibits oxidative metabolism leading to lactic acid accumulation. Ethylene glycol metabolism produces both oxalic acid and formic acid—the latter leading to lactic acid accumulation. Since ethylene glycol and methyl alcohol require alcohol dehydrogenase in their degradation ethyl alcohol may be therapeutic by tieing up the alcohol dehydrogenase and preventing its action on these two potentially toxic alcohols.

Salicylates first produce a respiratory alkalosis followed by a metabolic acidosis. The former is more characteristic of adults—the latter is more common in children. Salicylic acid is buffered by HCO_3^- whereas HCO_3^- is replaced by salicylates, ketones, and other organic anions. Therapy includes $NaHCO_3$ to maintain the blood pH and keep salicylate in the ionized form, which is less permeable across cell membranes than the unionized form.

An alkaline urine may enhance renal excretion by maintaining the urinary salicylate in the less permeable ionized form and decreasing tubular reabsorption.

Acute and chronic renal failure are associated with metabolic acidosis. In acute renal failure and most cases of chronic renal failure the acidosis is characterized by an increase in the anion gap due to the retention of normally filtered acid anions, such as SO_4^{2-}, PO_4^{2-}, and organic acid anions. The hydrogen ions associated with these anions are buffered by extracellular HCO_3^- lowering its concentration. The $[HCO_3^-]$ would normally be maintained by increased renal HCO_3^- production but the decrease in functioning nephrons diminishes the quantity of NH_3 production so that insufficient HCO_3^- can be replaced to maintain acid–base homeostasis. Since titratable acid secretion is dependent on a limited amount of filtered phosphate it cannot adequately compensate for the loss of NH_3 production. One of the purposes of the high caloric, low protein diets used in renal failure is an attempt to decrease protein cababolism and minimize the production of these acids.

Hyperchloremic acidosis is sometimes seen in patients with chronic renal failure and mild azotemia. It usually occurs in patients with interstitial nephritis and may indicate the presence of dehydration and need for $NaHCO_3$ (27). In patients with diabetes mellitus, it may be associated with hyperkalemia and hypoaldosteronism.

The acidosis of chronic renal failure is buffered by the usual intracellular and extracellular buffers and secondary respiratory aklalosis. Despite the quantitative limitations of these buffer mechanisms, the continued daily production of fixed acid and progressive loss of nephron function, the serum $[HCO_3^-]$ usually stabilizes at approximately 12–18 mmoles/liter. Recent studies indicate that this is due in large degree to buffering by bone carbonate which has as its secondary effect a loss of bone calcium resulting in osteopenia and osteomalacia (19).

Hyperchloremic acidosis can result when gastrointestinal HCO_3^- is lost, exogenous HCl is added to the body or renal HCO_3^- losses occur with relatively good glomerular function.

The losses associated with diarrhea, biliary or pancreatic fistula, and small bowel drainage are rich in Na^+ and K^+ HCO_3^- resulting in acidosis and dehydration. The $[Cl^-]$ increases because of the "contraction" of the extracellular fluid around the Cl^- whereas the kidney is stimulated by the hypovolemia to increase proximal Na^+ reabsorption. The reabsorbed Na^+ is accompanied by Cl^- in preference to H^+ exchange because of the lack of HCO_3^- in the glomerular filtrate to buffer secreted H^+. The compensatory low PCO_2 will also inhibit H^+ secretion.

In ureterosigmoidostomy, HCO_3^- losses are excessive because of active

HCO_3 secretion by the colonic mucosa. Urea is broken down by colonic bacteria to form NH_3, which is absorbed as NH_4Cl and converted to urea and HCl in the liver. Hyperchloremic acidosis in patients with ureteroileostomies usually indicates stasis of urine in the ileal loop allowing a similar process to occur as noted in ureterosigmoidostomies. Frequent evacuation may improve the hyperchloremic acidosis in ureterosigmoidostomies whereas surgical correction including shortening of the ileal loop or relieving stomal obstruction may be necessary in ureteroileostomies.

Cholestyramine is an ion-exchange resin used to prevent the intestinal absorption of bile acids. It also absorbs HCO_3^- in exchange for Cl^- and may lead to hyperchloremic metabolic acidosis in patients with renal insufficiency who cannot replace the HCO_3^-.

Renal tubular acidosis can be divided into proximal (II) and distal (I) types.

Proximal (II) RTA may be primary or secondary to many causes including chronic renal disease, Fanconi and Fanconi-like syndromes, Sjögren's syndrome, hyperparathyroidism, heavy metal or toxic damage to the proximal tubules, carbonic anhydrase inhibitors, nephrotic syndrome, multiple myeloma, and outdated tetracycline. It results from a limitation in H^+ secretion by the proximal tubules so that normal amounts of filtered HCO_3^- exceed the absorptive capacity producing an alkaline urine containing HCO_3^-. When plasma $[HCO_3^-]$ is reduced, the limited proximal secretion of H^+ is sufficient to reabsorb most of the filtered HCO_3^- and the urine becomes acid and bicarbonate free. Proximal PTA may be associated with aminoaciduria, glycosuria, phosphaturia, and uricosuria indicating failure of other reabsorptive functions of the proximal tubule.

Distal (I) RTA may be primary or inherited and secondary to interstitial renal disease, hyperglobulinemias, amphotericin B or lithium distal nephron damage, amyloidosis, medullary sponge kidney, cirrhosis, and renal transplantation. It is characterized by an inability of the distal tubule to develop a maximal urine to blood H^+ gradient of 1000 to 1.* Therefore, all of the HCO_3^- delivered distally (15% of filtered HCO_3^-) cannot be reabsorbed and HCO_3^- is always present in the final urine. Urine pH cannot go below 5.5 even after the ingestion of 0.1 gm/kg of NH_4Cl.

In both types of RTA the loss of HCO_3^- results in Na^+ and K^+ loss since the increased Na^+ excreted with HCO_3^- enhances Na^+-K^+ exchange in the distal tubule. The exchange is enhanced by the $2°$ hyperaldosteronism resulting from the hypovolemic state. In proximal RTA these $Na^+ + K^+$

_____
* Minimal distal urine pH is 4.4 whereas blood has a pH of 7.4.

losses cease when the plasma $[HCO_3^-]$ drops below the decreased proximal reabsorptive threshold. Although the Na^+ and K^+ losses in distal RTA are continuous they do not reach the magnitude attained in the proximal form. The chronic acidosis in distal RTA results in loss of bone calcium: hypercalciuria, nephrocalcinosis and nephrolithiasis, and osteomalacia. In proximal RTA the tubular losses of amino acids and a decreased proximal reabsorption of filtered citrate chelate the urine calcium preventing nephrocalcinosis and nephrolithiasis.

The treatment of distal RTA is $Na^+HCO_3^-$ or $Na^+- K^+$ citrate given as Shohl's solution. This will completely reverse the bone disease and prevent further renal damage. Adults with proximal RTA and $[HCO_3^-]$ greater than 18 mmoles/liter do not need therapy whereas children may need large amounts of Na^+ and $K^+HCO_3^-$ as well as vitamin D and oral phosphate therapy to compensate for increased renal losses of phosphate. Mild volume depletion with diuretics may decrease the requirement of alkali therapy in proximal RTA by enhancing proximal $NaHCO_3^-$ reabsorption.

Hyperalimentation can produce hyperchloremic acidosis by loading the patient with organic cations, such as lysine HCl, in excess of organic anions, such as Na acetate. Lysine HCl is converted by the liver to protein and HCl.

Dilutional hyperchloremic acidosis can be caused by infusing saline into the patient and diluting the plasma $[HCO_3^-]$. Although the plasma $[dCO_2]$ and $[H_2CO_3]$ are also reduced the cerebral respiratory center compensates for the decrease in $[dCO_2]$ by a slight decrease in ventilation to maintain the plasma CO_2 concentration. The brain reacts more slowly to the decrease in plasma $[HCO_3^-]$ because of the relative impermeability of the blood–brain barrier to HCO_3^-.

Acute metabolic acidosis is less well tolerated than chronic metabolic acidosis. It may cause a decrease in ventricular function and peripheral vascular resistance resulting in hypotension, shock, and pulmonary edema. The goal in therapy is to recognize and correct the underlying disturbance and bring the blood pH to reasonable levels. This can usually be accomplished by bringing the serum $[HCO_3^-]$ to 15 mEq/liter with $NaHCO_3^-$. Since approximately 50% of fixed acid buffering is intracellular, replacement can be calculated by subtracting the serum $[HCO_3^-]$ from 15 mEq/liter multiplying the difference by the extracellular H_2O (20% of body weight) and doubling the product.* The replacement of fluid can be given over 12–24 h with the rate of administration based on fre-

---

* In some patients with chronic metabolic acidosis the intracellular buffering of H^+ is greater than 50% and larger amounts of HCO_3^- replacement may be required (13).

quent measurement of acid–base parameters. Too rapid administration of $NaHCO_3^-$ may result in a respiratory alkalosis since HCO_3^- penetrates the blood–brain barrier slowly and the patient may continue to hyperventilate for some time even though the blood pH has returned to normal.

$NaHCO_3^-$ is the preferred salt for the correction of metabolic acidosis since Na lactate may not be adequately metabolized. In the presence of cardiac or renal failure the sodium (osmolar) load required to deliver sufficient amounts of HCO_3^- may be prohibitive. These patients cannot be effectively treated with Tris buffer [tris(hydroxymethyl)aminomethane] since the osmolar load is similar to that of $NaHCO_3^-$ and hemodialysis or peritoneal dialysis may be required (16).

D. Metabolic Alkalosis

Metabolic alkalosis results from a gain of base or loss of fixed acid from the body. It is characterized by an increase in $[HCO_3^-]$ and a tendency to decrease $[H^+]$ in the blood. The buffer mechanisms that resist the change in $[H^+]$ are tissue buffering, a decrease in respiration, and a loss of HCO_3^- by the kidney.

Under normal conditions the kidneys have a high capacity to excrete HCO_3^-, therefore, the maintenance of an elevated blood $[HCO_3^-]$ indicates the persistance of initiating mechanisms or an interference with the renal loss of HCO_3^-. These interfering factors include an enhanced proximal tubular Na^+-H^+ exchange due to a decrease in third factor,* a lack of Cl^- in the glomerular filtrate, and an increased distal tubular H^+ secretion due to hyperaldosteronism and hypokalemia.

The signs and symptoms of metabolic alkalosis include mental confusion, obtundation, neuromuscular irritability, cardiac arrythmias, and hypotension. These abnormalities may be related to associated hypovolemia, hypokalemia, hypocalcemia, and hypoxia. Alkalosis depresses respiration by decreasing stimulation of the peripheral chemoreceptors and medullary respiratory center. It also acutely shifts the oxyhemoglobin dissociation curve to the left making less oxygen available to the tissues.

It is useful to characterize the clinical conditions associated with metabolic alkalosis by the urinary $[Cl^-]$. A low urinary $[Cl^-]$ is found in those conditions where the elevated plasma $[HCO_3^-]$ is maintained by an increased proximal Na^+-H^+ exchange due to a decreased third factor ef-

---

* Third factor may be a hormone, which inhibits tubular sodium reabsorption, but more likely is the effect of physical factors. A decrease in hydrostatic pressure or an increase in oncotic pressure in the peritubular vessels favors sodium reabsorption whereas an increase in hydrostatic pressure or a decrease in oncotic pressure favors natriuresis.

TABLE VII

Causes of Metabolic Alkalosis

Urine $(Cl^-) < 10$ mEq/liter	Urine $(Cl^-) > 20$ mEq/liter
Hyperemesis	Primary hyperaldosteronism
Gastric suction	DOCA excess
Chloride rich diarrhea	Cushing's syndrome
Diuretics (late)	Licorice
Posthypercapneic alkalosis	Severe K^+ depletion
	Diuretics (early)
	Bartter's syndrome
Miscellaneous	
Milk alkali syndrome	
Recovery phase of ketoacidosis or lactic acidosis	
Hypoparathyroidism	
Hypercalcemia	

fect. A "high" urinary $[Cl^-]$ is found in conditions of high mineralcorticoid activity and/or hypokalemia without a proximal salt retaining state. (See Table VII)

Hyperemesis and gastric suction entails a loss of HCl from the body. Since the hydrogen ions are derived from H_2CO_3 these losses result in an elevation of blood $[HCO_3^-]$ whereas the Cl^- loss lowers blood $[Cl^-]$:

$$CO_2 + H_2O \xrightarrow{\text{CA}} H_2CO_3 \longleftrightarrow H^+ + HCO_3^- \qquad (14)$$

As blood $[HCO_3^-]$ exceeds the renal threshold HCO_3^- is lost in the urine with associated cations such as Na^+ and K^+ resulting in dehydration and hypokalemia. Dehydration decreases effective blood volume and enhances proximal Na^+ reabsorption. To maintain electroneutrality Na^+ reabsorption is linked to Cl^- reabsorption, but the lack of Cl^- causes the Na^+ reabsorption to be balanced by H^+ secretion, which results in increased HCO_3^- reabsorption and maintains the high blood $[HCO_3^-]$.

Chloride-rich diarrhea associated with congenital chloridorrhea and villous adenoma of the colon contains more Cl^- than HCO_3^- and results in hypovolemia with renal effects as described above.

The chronic use of the powerful loop diuretics can result in hypovolemia and choloride loss. Since these diuretics do not block the proximal tubular reabsorption of Na^+, the combination of hypovolemia and low-filtered Cl^- results in increased proximal $Na^+–H^+$ exchange and maintains the alkalosis.

Posthypercapneic alkalosis occurs as the aftermath of respiratory acidosis frequently associated with heart failure. During respiratory acidosis the increase pCO_2 selectively stimulates renal tubular Na^+–H^+ exchange and HCO_3^- reabsorption in excess of Cl^- reabsorption. The resulting Cl^- loss combined with the use of salt-restricted diets and diuretics causes hypochloremia and a further decrease in effective blood volume. These maintain the proximal HCO_3^- reabsorption after the respiratory acidosis has been corrected. At this stage the low [Cl^-] in the glomerular filtrate and the enhanced proximal absorption of available Na^+Cl^- results in a low urinary [Cl^-].

Primary hyperaldosteronism, DOCA excess, and Cushing's syndrome represent states of mineralcorticoid excess whereas the glycyrrhizic acid derived from licorice mimics aldosterone in its tubular effects. The increased circulating blood volume resulting from mineralcorticoid stimulated distal tubular Na^+ reabsorption causes a "third factor" proximal tubular effect, which decreases proximal tubular Na^+Cl^- reabsorption. Much of the Na^+ delivered distally is reabsorbed in exchange for K^+ and H^+ by the activated mineralcorticoid mechanism whereas the Cl^- escapes into the urine. The excessive H^+ and K^+ secretion results in increased HCO_3^- addition to the blood and hypokalemia.

Severe K^+ depletion produces extracellular metabolic alkalosis by causing H^+ to shift intracellularly and increasing H^+ secretion in both the proximal and distal nephron. Hypokalemia enhances NH_3 secretion, which also increases HCO_3^- formation. It may block Cl^- reabsorption in the distal nephron enchancing H^+ secretion and HCO_3^- formation while increasing the urine [Cl^-] (12).

The potent loop diuretics, such as furosemide and ethacrynic acid, block Cl^- reabsorption in the loop of Henle and probably also in the cortical collecting tubule segment. The latter favors H^+ and K^+ secretion because of increased luminal negativity. This results in increased blood [HCO_3^-], hypokalemia, and an increased urine [Cl^-] until the diuretic produces hypovolemia.

Bartter's syndrome is a rare disorder, which may be due to a renal tubular Cl^- leak obligating losses of Na^+ and K^+. It is associated with increased renin and aldosterone secretion, which may be due to increased renal prostaglandin production. Treatment consists of K^+ replacement, spironolactone to block aldosterone and Indocin to block prostaglandin production (5).

Milk alkali syndrome results when patients with peptic ulcer disease chronically ingest large amounts of milk, $CaCO_3$, and $NaHCO_3$. This can produce renal insufficiency due to nephrocalcinosis while the continued ingestion of absorbable alkali can exceed the damaged kidney's ability to excrete HCO_3^-, producing metabolic alkalosis.

Both hypoparathyroidism and nonparathyroid hypercalcemia can increase tubular H^+ secretion resulting in increased HCO_3^- reabsorption and mild metabolic alkalosis.

The treatment of metabolic alkalosis is most successful if the initiating factors can be discontinued and the maintenance factors corrected. NaCl therapy is usually indicated for the low urine $[Cl^-]$ group whereas salt restriction, aldosterone antagonists, and KCl therapy may be required for the higher urine $[Cl^-]$ group. K^+ replacement therapy requires correction of the serum $[K^+]$ for intracellular shifts induced by the pH change.*

If the kidneys are damaged they may not be able to excrete the accumulated HCO_3^- despite correction of hypovolemia and Cl^- or K^+ deficits. This problem may be complicated by the patient's inability to tolerate the required amounts of Na^+ because of renal and cardiac failure. Acidifying salts such as NH_4Cl, arginine HCl, and HCL have been utilized in this situation (NH_4Cl is contraindicated in the presence of liver disease). $0.15\ N$ HCl can be safely administered through a central venous catheter (1).

Since approximately one-third of an alkali load is buffered intracellularly, the amount of acidifying solution required can be calculated by multiplying the extracellular $[HCO_3^-]$ excess by $\frac{3}{2}$.

$$60 \text{ kg man with } [HCO_3^-] = 36 \text{ mEq/liter}$$
$$36 - 24 = 12 \text{ mEq/liter excess}$$
$$12 \text{ mEq/liter} \times 12 \text{ liters (ECW)} = 144 \text{ mEqs}$$
$$144 \times 3/2 = 216 \text{ mEqs (acid requirement)}$$

(15)

If the alkalotic patient is overhydrated with renal failure, it may be necessary to dialyze him with high chloride solutions to remove the excess HCO_3^- and provide the Cl^- replacement (31).

E. Mixed Acid–Base Disorders

The common mixed acid–base disorders include:

1. Respiratory acidosis and metabolic alkalosis as seen in patients with chronic respiratory acidosis who receive excessive amounts of diuretics. The findings may include a $[HCO_3^-]$ inappropriately high for the pCO_2, a low serum $[K^+]$, and an increased alveolar–arterial oxygen gradient.

---

* A guide for the correction of serum $[K^+]$ when pH is altered is based on the expected extracellular shift of K^+ in metabolic acidosis and intracellular shift in metabolic alkalosis. $\uparrow 0.1$ pH = $\downarrow 0.7$ mEq/liter (K^+). Each mEq/liter decrease in corrected $[K^+]$ down to $3.0 = 100–200$ mEq deficit. Each mEq/liter decrease in corrected $[K^+]$ below $3.0 = 200–400$ mEq;liter further deficit (26). Organic acids may be less effective in elevating serum $[K^+]$ than inorganic acids (22).

2. Respiratory acidosis and metabolic acidosis as seen in patients with acute cardiorespiratory arrest. The metabolic acidosis is associated with lactic acidosis. Therapy includes the correction of hypoxia and the administration of $NaHCO_3$.
3. Respiratory alkalosis and metabolic acidosis as seen in patients with salicylate poisoning or renal failure superimposed on the hyperventilation of hepatic failure. Salicylates stimulate the respiratory center but also produce a high anion gap acidosis.

The presence of a mixed disorder may be suspected from the history and physical. Further clues include a normal pH despite abnormal $[HCO_3^-]$ and pCO_2, an inappropriate secondary response for a simple disturbance (Table II), an increased anion gap in a patient without apparent metabolic acidosis, an increased alveolar–arterial oxygen gradient in a patient with hypoventilation apparently due to metabolic alkalosis. The serum $[K^+]$ may be helpful since it will tend to increase in a simple acidosis and decrease in a simple alkalosis.*

REFERENCES

1. Abouna, G. M., Veuzey, P. C., and Terry, D. B. (1974). *Surgery* **75,** 194–198.
2. Albert, M. S., Dell, R. B., and Winters, R. W. (1967). *Ann. Intern. Med.* **66,** 312.
3. Arbus, G. S., Herbert, L. A., Levesque, P. R., Etsen, B. E., and Schwartz, W. B. (1969). *N. Engl. J. Med.* **280,** 117.
4. Astrup, P., Jorgensen, K., Siggaard-Andersen, O., and Engel, E. (1960). *Lancet* **1,** 1035–1039.
5. Bardgette, J., and Stein, J. H. (1979). *In* "Pathophysiology of Bartter's Syndrome in Acid-Base and Potassium Homeostasis" (B. M. Brenner and J. H. Stein, eds.), pp. 269–297. Churchill Livingstone, New York.
6. Brackett, N. C., Jr., Cohen, J. J., and Schwartz, W. B. (1965). *N. Engl. J. Med.* **276,** 6.
7. Brackett, N. C., Jr., Wingo, C. F., Muren, O., and Salnao, J. T. (1969). *N. Engl. J. Med.* **280,** 124.
8. Cohen, J. J., and Madias, N. E. (1978). *In* "Acid-Base Disturbance of Respiratory Origin in Acid-Base and Potassium Homeostasis," (B. M. Brenner and J. H. Stein, eds.), pp. 137–167. Churchill Livingstone, New York.
9. Davenport, H. W. (1975). "The ABC of Acid-Base Chemistry," 6th. Ed. Univ. of Chicago Press, Chicago, Illinois.
10. Fagen, T. J. (1973). *N. Engl. J. Med.* **288,** 915.
11. Fulop, M. (1976). *N. Y. State J. Med.* **76,** 19–22.
12. Garella, S., Chazan, J. A., and Cohen, V. V. (1970). *Ann. Intern. Med.* **73,** 31–38.
13. Garella, S., Dana, C. L., and Chazan, J. A. (1973). *N. Engl. J. Med.* **289,** 121–126.

* This is more pertinent to metabolic than to respiratory disorders because a low (HCO_3^-) and low pH are complimentary in promoting extracellular shifts of K^+ while the opposite is true of high (HCO_3^-) and an increased pH.

14. Gennari, F. J., Goldstein, M. B., and Schwartz, W. B. (1972). *J. Clin. Invest.* **51**, 1722.
15. Huber, G. L. (1978). "Arterial Blood Gas and Acid-Base Physiology in Current Concepts." The Upjohn Company, Kalamazoo, Michigan.
16. Kaehny, W. D. (1976). *In* "Renal and Electrolyte Disorders" (R. J. Schrier, ed.), pp. 79–121. Little, Brown, Boston, Massachusetts.
17. Kassirer, J. P., and Bleich, H. L. (1965). *N. Engl. J. Med.* **272**, 1067–1068.
18. Clark, L. C., Jr. (1956). *Trans. Am. Soc. Art. Int. Organs* **2**, 41–45.
19. Lemann, J., Jr., Litzow, R., and Lennon, E. J. (1966). *J. Clin. Invest.* **45**, 1608.
20. Monge , C. C., Lozano, R., and Carcelen, C. (1964). *J. Clin. Invest.* **43**, 2303.
21. Narins, R. G. (1978). *In* "Renal Acidosis in Acid-Base and Potassium Homeostasis" (B. M. Brenner and J. H. Stein, eds.), pp. 30–65. Churchill Livingstone, New York.
22. Oster, J. R., Perez, G. O., and Vaamonde, C. A. (1978). *Am. J. Physiol.* **235**, F345.
23. Pitts, R. F. (1974). "Physiology of the Kidney and Body Fluids," 3rd. Ed. pp. 189–191. Year Book Pub., Chicago, Illinois.
24. Saltzman, H., Heyman, A., and Sieker, H. (1963). *N. Engl. J. Med.* **268**, 1431.
25. Schwartz, W. B., and Relman, A. S. (1963). *N. Engl. J. Med.* 1382–1388.
26. Scribner, B. H., and Burnell, J. M. (1956). *Metabolism* **5**, 468.
27. Seldin, D. W., Carter, N. W., and Rector, F. C., Jr., (1971). *In* "Diseases of the Kidney" (M. B. Strauss and L. G. Welt, eds.), pp. 227–231. Little, Brown, Boston, Massachusetts.
28. Severinghaus, J. W. (1965). "Blood Gas Concentration in Handbook of Physiology," Section 3, Respiration, Vol 2, pp. 1425. Williams and Wilkins, Baltimore, Maryland.
29. Siggaard-Andersen, O. (1963). *Scand. J. Clin. Lab. Invest.* **15**, 211–217.
30. Singer, R. B. (1948). *Am. J. Med. Sci.* **221**, 199–210.
31. Swartz, R. D., Rubin, J. E., Brown, R. S., Jager, H. M., and Steinman, T. I. (1977). *Ann. Intern. Med.* **86**, 52–55.
32. Van Slyke, D. D., and Neill, J. M. (1924). *Int. J. Biol. Chem.* **61**, 523.
33. Winters, R. W., Engel, K., and Dell, R. B. (1969). "Respiratory Alkalosis in Acid-Base Physiology in Medicine," pp. 253. The London Company of Cleveland and Radiometer A/S of Copenhagen.

6

Autoimmune Disease

GLORIA A. MARCANTUONO

CLINICAL BIOCHEMISTRY
Contemporary Theories and Techniques, Vol. 1

I. INTRODUCTION

Immunology is the study of the physiological mechanisms by which animals defend themselves against microorganisms and malignant cell formation. As with all new languages, one must become familiar with the terminology used to explain the complex mechanisms involved in the immune response. The immunosurveillance system can be compared to an orchestral arrangement, with each component intertwining harmonies at both the humoral and cellular levels. The first part of this chapter will serve as a guide to the new immunologic concepts put forth during the last 20 years, a period that can be referred to as the renaissance of modern-day immunology.

II. GENERAL REVIEW OF THE IMMUNE RESPONSE

A. Antigenicity

All things in nature will not respond unless there is a stimulus, and the immune system is no exception. An antigen is a "nonself" macromolecule that provokes an immune response when introduced into the tissues of animals. The response can be at a humoral (antibody) or cellular level. Paul Ehrlick (35a), in his principle of "horror autotoxicus" (fear of self-poisoning) recognized the fact that antigens must be foreign in order to elicit a specific immune response. He proposed that antigenic components normally present in the peripheral bloodstream of an animal cannot be antigenic for that animal. He further concluded that if this were not the case we would soon synthesize antibodies to our own cellular components leading to a condition that would surely end in certain death. Consequently, the body has devised a fail safe mechanism that minimizes autoantibody formation. Ehrlick's concept to this day, remains essentially sound!

B. Cellular Cooperation—B Cells, T Cells, and Macrophages

In the early 1900s, Ehrlick (35b) also proposed the, now famous, side chain theory. His was one of the first major hypotheses of humoral or antibody-mediated immunity. Metchnikoff (78) belonged to an alternate school of thought and proposed the cellular theory of immunity. Today, evidence from experimental animal models and studies on patients with congenital immunodeficiencies, indicates that both theories were indeed correct.

Cells participating in the immune response can be divided into two distinct lymphocytic populations. Thymus gland processed T cells and bone marrow derived B cells[48].

When sensitized by nonself antigen, T cells are capable of mounting a cell-mediated response that affords protection against microorganisms and malignant cell formation. Through an elaborate system of signals at the cellular level, macrophages absorb and concentrate antigen on their cell membranes. A "super antigen" is thus presented to the activated T lymphocyte and culminates in T cell proliferation and ultimately effective cell mediated response. T cells do not secrete antibody but cooperate with B cells, which in turn produce antibodies. Investigators have divided T lymphocytes into subsets. The major subsets include (1) T helper cells (91)—required for antibody production and (2) T suppressor cells, (74) responsible for regulating antibody production by B cells.

The second major lymphocyte population is comprised of the B cells or the mediators of humoral response. These cells, unlike T cells, mature in the bone marrow or possibly the lining of the intestinal tract or spleen[48]. When B cells are stimulated by antigen they proliferate and differentiate into plasma cells, which are the major source of highly specific antibody. B cells may be stimulated directly, by antigens, or indirectly, by helper T cells.

Still another class of cells are referred to as killer cells (92b). They are cytotoxic *in vitro* to tumor cells. In cell culture systems, killer cells seem to be bound by specific antibody and destroy target cells on a one to one basis.

The macrophage (30) is a specialized phagocytotic cell that collaborates with T lymphocytes. The mechanisms by which this mononuclear cell operates in maintaining the purity of the internal environment is intriguing. The macrophage is first attracted to a primed or sensitized T cell via a soluble chemical substance termed chemotactic factor. It is then immobilized in the T cells vicinity by a lymphokine (an alternate soluble chemical substance) termed Macrophage Inhibiting Factor, whereupon it is programmed for final activation and killing function. The armed, or "angry," macrophage (55) undergoes a unique metamorphosis. Its plasma membrane becomes enlarged and ruffled, phagocytotic capabilities are greatly enhanced, and lysosomal enzyme production is increased. The armed macrophage has incredible nonspecific killing ability and appears to play a crucial role in antigen and tumor destruction as well as antibody synthesis.

The complement system (80b) is yet another integral component of the immune response. It is an enzymatic system made up of serum proteins, and is activated by antibody–antigen complex formation. Complement is needed for a myriad of immunologic mechanisms, such as chemotaxis, phagocytosis, opsonization, and immune cytolysis.

C. Antibody Structure and Function

A functional definition of an antibody is, simply, a serum protein synthesized by an animal in response to an antigenic stimulus. Serum proteins can be separated by analytical ultracentrifugation in 19 S (900,000 molecular weight, mainly IgM globulin and α-2-macroglobulin), 7 S (150,000 molecular weight, mainly IgG and IgA globulin), and 4 S (60,000 molecular weight, mainly albumin) (92b).

1. Immunoglobulin G

In 1972, a joint Nobel Prize in physiology and medicine was awarded to Edelman at the Rockefeller University and Porter at Oxford University for their fascinating studies that unraveled the complex structure of IgG (5). Porter (5,90) used an enzymatic approach and treated rabbit IgG with papain. He discovered two fragments which he termed Fab and Fc respectively. The Fab fragment retained the antigen binding capacity, while the Fc fragment crystallized easily. Edelman tried an alternate approach and utilized disulfide bond reduction. He discovered that the IgG molecule was comprised of two polypeptide chains termed heavy (H) chains (55,000 molecular weight) and light (L) chains (22,000 molecular weight). Porter and Edelman's elegant experiments resulted in the construction of a symmetrical four peptide model consisting of two heavy and two light chains held together by interchain disulfide bonds. The heavy and light chains in the Fab fragments were further divided into constant and variable regions. In addition, the amino acids between the Fab and Fc fragments were called hinge peptides and were found to aid in molecular flexibility (55). Figure 1.

Generally, the intact IgG molecule consists of one Fc portion (involved in complement fixation, skin fixation or placental transfer) and two Fab portions (involved in antigen binding). All IgG molecules are bivalent and contain two antigen binding sites directed against the same antigenic determinant; 75–85% of all antibodies belong to this class of immunoglobulins. They are also involved in the secondary immune response (92b).

2. Immunoglobulin A

Immunoglobulin A (55, 115) is a basic four chain structure similar to IgG. This molecule has a tendency to form polymers spontaneously and may appear as an 11 S dimer. Secretory IgA, the major antibody found in external secretions, is composed of two IgA molecules and a "secretory piece" linked together by a unique joining J chain. The function of the latter is to hold two molecules together, resulting in four antigen binding sites. Immunoglobulin A represents 13% of all serum immunoglobulins.

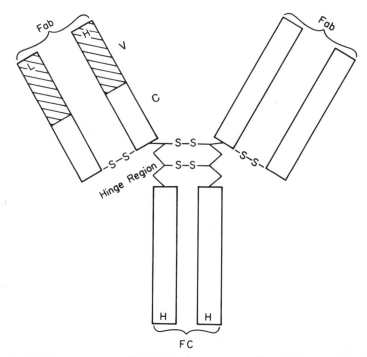

Fig. 1. Fab, fragment antigen binding; Fc, fragment crystallized; H, heavy chain; L, light chain; V, variable region; C, constant region; S—S, disulfide bonds.

Its major function is to defend external surfaces against bacterial invasion. It is, therefore, found in saliva, sweat, tears, colostrum, and secretions of the lung and gastrointestinal tract.

3. Immunoglobulin M

Immunoglobulin M (92b) exists as a pentamer of the basic four chain antibody molecule. The five four-chain units are held together by disulfide bonds and a J chain. IgM is a 19 S globulin with a molecular weight of 800,000–900,000 and is phylogenetically the most primitive immunoglobulin. Due to their high molecular weight, IgM immunoglobulins are excellent agglutinating and cytolytic agents, and are the mediators of the primary immune response.

4. Immunoglobulin E

Immunoglobulin E (92b), the most recently discovered antibody, is synthesized predominantly by plasma cells in the lamina propria of gastrointestinal and respiratory epithelium. It is an 8 S (200,000 molecular weight) immunoglobulin and is present in normal serum at very low concentrations (300 ng/ml). IgE has been shown to be responsible for skin sensitization and allergic responses (59). This antibody demonstrates the remarkable capability of binding to mast cells in the skin and respiratory tract. Contact with antigen (pollen, dust, animal dander, etc.) leads to the degradation of mast cells with subsequent histamine release. Serum IgE levels are markedly elevated in patients with allergic asthma, hay fever, and parasitic infections. Recently, it has been suggested that IgE may be crucially involved in the immune response to malignant cell formation (94).

5. Immunoglobulin D

Immunoglobulin D (92b) has been found on the surface of lymphocytes and may function as an antigen receptor. It is a 7 S antibody with a molecular weight of 185,000 and comprises 1% of the total serum immunoglobulins.

III. IMMUNOPATHOLOGY OF AUTOIMMUNE MULTISYSTEM DISEASE

In most normal individuals, there exists a recognition or tolerance of "SELF"—that is a fail-safe mechanism that prohibits the destruction of body constituents. In autoimmune disease, there is a breakdown of this fail-safe mechanism. Harmful sequelae develop. Body constituents are deemed foreign, complement is activated, humoral and cellular devices are set into motion, and a state of "horror autotoxicus" ensues.

The spectrum of autoimmune disease ranges from organ specific such as Hashimoto's thyroiditis to nonorgan specific or multisystem disease such as systemic lupus erythematosus.

A. Multisystem Disease

1. Systemic Lupus Erythematosus

Systemic lupus erythematosus (SLE) is considered by many investigators to be the prototype of autoimmune disorders. It is a chronic inflammatory hypersensitivity disease primarily affecting young women. Its major characteristic pathologic changes occur in the vascular system, since collagen, which serves as a mordant for capillaries and small blood vessels, is ultimately destroyed. SLE is classified as a multisystem dis ease because it affects the skin, joints, serous membranes, eyes, kidneys, and central nervous system. In fulminant SLE, the glomerulobasement membrane of the kidneys and CNS are severely damaged, which tends to be the major cause of death.

The term lupus erythematosus, which in Latin means red wolf, was first used by the French dermatologist Pierre Louis Cazenave (32c). He described the dermatologic manifestations as erythematous ulcerations about the face. The disease was first thought to be a malignancy of the skin, (resembling the bite of a wolf) and was later listed as a tuberculous disease. It remained under this classification until the early 1900s.

In 1872, a Viennese dermatologist Moritz Kaposi (32c) was the first to describe SLE as a serious acute often fatal disease. He further differentiated discoid lupus (primarily involving skin) from the systemic form, and described the classic facial lesions as butterfly in shape.

In the early 1900s various internists and pathologists collaborated in an attempt to understand the complex mechanisms involved in this disease process. They proposed that the glomerulus was the site of antibody–antigen precipitation and considered this phenomenon the underlying cause of SLE nephropathy. Today, investigators have found that the development of *SLE nephropathy is dependent upon the deposition of circulating immune complexes* within the glomerular basement membrane (63b). Unanue and Dixon (121) challenged experimental animals with purified glomerular basement membrane material in Freund's complete adjuvant—severe nephritis developed. Lerner and Dixon (69) transferred ovine (sheep) experimental allergic glomerulonephritis (EAG) with serum. Experiments like these led to a more complete understanding of the immunopathologic mechanisms involved in autoimmune glomerulonephritis.

2. Lupus Erythematosus (LE) Cell Test

The discovery of the LE cell by Hargraves (54) gave impetus to further immunologic investigation of SLE patients. With repeated testing, a circulating peripheral bloodstream autoantibody can be detected in about 90% of all SLE patients (32b). This phenomenon is a highly characteristic feature of the disease and is referred to as the LE cell factor (8) (32b). The LE cell factor has been found to be an IgG 7 S antibody with specific reactivity against the DNA–histone complex. This complex comprises the major nucleoprotein component of all cell nuclei. (32b)

SLE sera containing the LE cell factor have the ability to react with extracted nucleoprotein in disrupted leukocytes. The damaged nucleus enlarges, producing a modification of the nuclear material and forms what is termed a hematoxylin body (32c). In the presence of complement, a portion of this basophilic homogeneous mass is phagocytized by intact poly-morphonuclear neutrophils (PMNs) and an LE cell is formed (32b). The clinical relevance of the LE cell test is a hotly debated subject. It has been reported to be positive in only 50–80% of all active cases of SLE and, therefore, has been discontinued in some clinical laboratories (86). Others, however, continue to rely heavily on the clinical significance of the LE cell prep when a diagnosis of SLE is suspected (125).

3. Clinical Significance of the Antinuclear Antibody Test

Antinuclear antibodies (ANA) consist of a heterogeneous group of au-toantibodies that react with various nuclear antigens (21). They are con-sistently found in the sera of patients with many types of autoimmune dis-ease manifestations. *In vitro,* ANA are not species specific since they react with nuclear components of different species. ANA usually belong to the IgG and IgM class of immunoglobulins but can also be of the IgA, IgE, or IgD classes.

In the early 1950s, Coons developed immunofluorescence (27b). This valuable *in vitro* technique was applied to the blood and tissues of SLE patients, (27a) and ultimately resulted in the formation of the indirect im-munofluorescent antinuclear antibody test (IIF-ANA). At present, it is the most widely used method for ANA detection and is the method of choice for screening purposes (21).

Other conventional immunologic methods such as complement fixa-tion, passive hemagglutination, radioimmunoassay, and latex fixation have been used to detect ANA. These methods have met with varying de-grees of success since they require purified antigens, sophisticated equip-ment, and at times, much technical expertise.

Many types of animal tissues can be used as antigenic substrates in the IIF-ANA assay. The reason for this is that ANA are not species- or organ-specific. Most systems employ mouse or rat liver sections. The principle of the IIF technique is as follows: tissue substrate (antigen) is overlayed with diluted serum (antibody) and incubated in a moist chamber for a specified amount of time. If ANA are present, they will bind to spe-cific antigenic sites. The unattached serum proteins are removed by washing with phosphate-buffered saline. A fluorescein isothiocyanate (FITC) labeled antihuman γ-globulin (antiantibody) is then applied to the tissue sections, and the slides are incubated once again. After another washing period, the sections are mounted in phosphate-buffered glycerol, coverslipped, and examined by fluorescence microscopy.

Several nuclear patterns have been reported (21, 10) and include:

1. Homogeneous—diffuse staining of the entire nucleus. This type of staining is caused by antibodies that are reactive to DNA nucleoprotein–histone complexes.
2. Peripheral or rim—staining of the nuclear membrane due to antibodies directed against double- and single-stranded DNA.
3. Speckled—dispersed specks of staining throughout the entire nucleus, due to antibodies directed against saline—extractable nucleoprotein (anti-SM and anti-RNP) antigen.
4. Nucleolar—staining of nucleolar membranes only, due to antibodies reactive with RNA nucleoprotein complexes.

ANA titer may not correlate with the clinical course of disease, but the various patterns seem to be associated with specific autoimmune disease states (21).

At present, the IIF-ANA test has supplanted the LE test (21), since the former will detect 95% of all active cases of SLE. The greatest value is that a negative result usually excludes a diagnosis of SLE.

The significance of a positive ANA test must be assessed in relationship to the patient's clinical history, age, sex, and other pertinent laboratory data. It must be stressed, however, that the demonstration of autoantibodies in a patient's serum simply indicates that an autoimmune reaction has taken place. This finding does not mean that autoantibodies are the mediators of autoimmune disease. Indeed, autoantibody production may be a result of pathologic changes (21).

4. Complement Levels

Complement levels can also be very valuable diagnostic tools (111) since they are often used to monitor the course of SLE. When exacerbation of the disease process occurs, complement is depleted from the circulating bloodstream and results in markedly depressed levels. In remission, however, complement levels return to normal.

TABLE I

ANA Interpretation

Pattern	Most often associated with
Homogeneous, high titer	Systemic lupus erythematosus
Homogeneous, low titer	Rheumatoid arthritis, age or drug related
Peripheral	Systemic lupus erythematosus
Speckled	Scleroderma, mixed connected tissue disease, Raynaud's syndrome, SLE
Nucleolar	Scleroderma

Courtesy of Donald R. Tourville, Zeus Scientific, Inc., Raritan, N.J.

5. Clinical Significance of n-DNA Antibodies

Anti-nDNA antibodies are found almost exclusively in the sera of SLE patients (1, 64, 110). When deposited as immune complexes in the glomerular basement membrane, these antibodies seem to be involved in the most fulminant form of renal pathogenesis (63a, 63c, 100, 131). Anti nDNA antibody titers generally appear to reflect the severity of the disease process since levels decline during periods of remission and increase during disease exacerbation (32d, 72).

Certain drugs can produce a disease syndrome indistinguishable from SLE. Some of the drugs that have been implicated include hydralazine, chlorpromazine, procanimide, and isoniazide (68). Furthermore, patients receiving these drugs can develop high ANA titers without producing classic SLE symptoms.

More than 400 cases of drug-induced SLE have been reported since the early 1940s (68). Much of the work on the mechanism of drug-induced SLE has been with hydralazine, an antihypertensive agent. Patients with hydralazine-induced SLE were found to have antibodies directed against the drug (53a). In tissue culture drug-induced SLE lymphocytes reacted against hydralazine whereas normal lymphocytes did not. The data collected from these studies suggests that the continual presence of the drug- and hydralazine-directed antibody may provide a stimulus for the development of SLE in a patient that has manifested ANA production.

For these reasons, it is therapeutically and diagnostically helpful to identify and quantitate nDNA levels. The nDNA assay is an extremely valuable test. By virtue of its specificity, it can differentially diagnose true SLE from drug-induced SLE.

Many techniques have been employed in the study of DNA levels. These include DNA spot test, (75) gel diffusion(41a), and the ammonium sulfate precipitation (36) or Farr assay. The initial methods were of little practical value, since standardization was often difficult. With the advent of radioimmunoassay, however, it was possible to measure nDNA antibodies much more accurately.

Recently, Aarden, de Groot, and Feltkamp (1) developed an IIF technique for the detection of antibodies against double-stranded native DNA. The kinetoplast of a hemoflagellate *Crithidia luciliae* consists of a single concentrated network of double-stranded nDNA, unassociated with histone, thus providing a simple substrate for the detection of nDNA antibodies.

If nDNA antibodies are present in a suspect SLE serum, they will bind to the kinetoplast of the *Crithidia luciliae* substrate. Rabbit antihuman γ-globulin labeled with FITC is then applied to the prepared slides. If the serum contains nDNA antibodies, the kinetoplasts will fluoresce a brilliant green when examined by fluorescence microscopy.

In a recent publication (24), the indirect immunofluorescent *Crithidia luciliae* (IIF-CL) assay was found to be as specific and sensitive as four other DNA antibody measurement methods. In addition, the IIF-CL test showed an increased frequency of positive tests in patients with active severe renal disease. A unique advantage of this technique was its ability to identify complement fixing nDNA antibodies. The authors correlated this finding with severe renal damage.

6. Direct Fluorescence Studies on Tissue Biopsies from SLE Patients

ANA combine with soluble antigen in the appropriate ratio to form immune complexes. These complexes localize in blood vessels in a widespread distribution and most always involve kidney glomeruli (63b).

SLE nephritis seems to be mediated by DNA–anti nDNA complex deposition in mesangial cells and along the glomerular basement membrane (65). Complex deposition is followed by complement activation (80a), which results in the release of chemotactic factors. PMNs are mobilized into the area and attach to the glomerular basement membrane where they release destructive lysosomal enzymes. The inflammatory insult spirals and leads to glomerular injury. This same mechanism elicits activation of the clotting mechanism and results in proliferation of glomerular epithelial and endothelial cells (117).

Renal biopsies from SLE patients are studied by the direct method of immunofluorescence staining. Cryostat kidney biopsy sections are overlayed with specific FITC-labeled anti-immunoglobulins and antiprotein components (anti IgG, IgM, IgA, C3, C4, and fibrinogen). The various sections are incubated in a moist chamber for a specified amount of time. The slides are then washed in phosphate-buffered saline to remove any unattached proteins, mounted, and examined by fluorescence microscopy.

In patients with characteristic SLE nephropathy, a "lumpy bumpy" (119) pattern is observed. This is caused by immune reactants scattered along the glomerular basement membrane in an irregular granular pattern.

B. Extractable Nuclear Antigen and Mixed Connective Tissue Disease

The diagnosis of autoimmune disease is often difficult, for it must be based on a combination of clinical, pathologic, and serologic criteria. Mixed connective tissue disease is a perplexing clinical entity that shares features of systemic lupus erythematosus, scleroderma, polymyositis, and Raynaud's phenomenon.

Gordon Sharp (101a) and other investigators (84, 98) have found this disorder to be marked by unusually high ANA titers with a specificity for nuclear ribonucleoprotein. This nuclear antigen was extracted from isolated cell nuclei in isotonic buffer, hence, the term extractable nuclear antigen. Through immunodiffusion studies (101b) it was revealed that ENA consisted of two definite antigens: (1) RNP—a nuclear ribonucleoprotein that is sensitive to ribonuclease (RNAse) and trypsin treatment and (2) the SM antigen, which is not. Both RNP and SM antigens are associated with speckled ANA staining patterns when IIF is employed.

Studies with both MCTD and SLE patients have revealed the following(12, 101c):

1. ENA has been demonstrated in 86% of those patients with SLE nephropathy who respond to therapy, but in only 8% of those who do not.
2. MCTD is also characterized by high ENA antibody titers.
3. 74% of patients with clinical features of MCTD have antibodies to RNAse-sensitive *ENA(RNP)*, and demonstrate speckled fluorescent ANA patterns.
4. Patients with antibodies to RNAse-resistant *ENA (SM)* also have speckled fluorescent ANA. 85% of these patients were found to have SLE.

Experimentally, ENA inhibits the *in vitro* precipitation and hemagglutination reactions between DNA and anti-DNA, therefore, suggesting that ENA may exert a protective effect by interfering with immune complex formation (101a). This hypothesis was tested in NZB/NZW mice, the experimental animal model of SLE (11). Preliminary results showed that renal disease in mice receiving weekly injections of ENA was significantly milder than in controls (101a).

C. Rheumatoid Arthritis

Rheumatoid arthritis (RA) is a chronic disease of the joints that affects the collagen substance of connective tissue. It generally involves diarthrodial joints and is characterized by inflammatory changes, atrophy and rarefaction of bones, transient stiffness and swelling with pain, tenderness and structural changes, which result in subcutaneous nodular formation.

Serologically, an IgM autoantibody is formed against antigenic determinants of an altered IgG molecule (66). This autoantibody is referred to as the rheumatoid factor (RF) (88). It has been suggested that infection may cause an alteration in joint tissue resulting in the formation of a neoantigen with continuous IgG production. The immunosurveillance system recognizes this altered IgG as foreign and synthesizes an IgM autoantibody (22). Rheumatoid factor is consistently demonstrated in the serous and synovial fluids of adults with established RA, but is seldom found in juvenile RA (45).

Qualitative and quantitative assessment of RF is accomplished by combining diluted sera with biologically inert carrier molecules coated with heat-denatured human IgG. Various carrier substances, such as latex particles and erythrocytes, have been used with great success. (93a, 104a, 122) The American Rheumatism Association has recently designated the latex tube method as the preferred technique (104b).

The serologic demonstration of RF, however, does not establish a diagnosis of RA, since this factor can be found in other unrelated disorders (130). Rather, the diagnosis should be more clinically determined by roentgenological findings, symptoms, and familial studies.

IV. IMMUNOPATHOLOGY OF AUTOIMMUNE ORGAN-SPECIFIC DISEASE

A. Immunopathology of Liver Disease

The concept of autoimmune liver disease is more speculative than definitive. To date, experimental autoimmune hepatitis cannot be induced by challenging animal models with purified liver extract (85a). Furthermore, liver-specific antibodies cannot be detected (85b).

Still, chronic liver syndromes do exist and seem to be mediated by underlying autoimmune phenomenon (31b). Most patients with autoimmune liver disease consistently demonstrate nonorgan-specific antibodies to subcellular organells and soluble proteins (117). These antibodies are directed against antigenic components shared by the liver and other organ systems.

Three distinct autoantibodies have been detected in patients with autoimmune liver syndromes. They include (1) antinuclear antibodies (ANA)—associated with all types of liver disorders (21); (2) smooth muscle antibodies (SMA) found in patients with chronic active hepatitis (60); and (3) mitochrondrial antibodies (MA) found in patients with primary biliary cirrhosis (62).

1. Association of Antinuclear Antibodies with Liver Disease

Antinuclear antibodies are the least diagnostically significant immunoglobulins detected in autoimmune liver maladies. These antibodies can be found in many nonliver-related disease states, in the normal elderly population, and in drug-induced syndromes (21).

Nevertheless, ANA were the first diagnostic markers used to differentiate autoimmune liver disease from prolonged cases of virally induced hepatitis and are detected in 75% of patients with chronic active hepatitis (31b). Generally, high ANA titers accompanied by persistently high SMA titers are considered important diagnostic features of lupoid or chronic active hepatitis.

2. Association of Smooth Muscle Antibodies with Chronic Active Hepatitis

Lupoid hepatitis, or chronic active hepatitis (CAH), is a chronic liver dysfunction primarily affecting young women. It is characterized by a progressive "piecemeal" necrosis of liver parenchymal cells. The lesions seem to be mediated by cellular infiltration of the portal tracts with subsequent proliferation of the bile ductules. Autoimmunity is evidenced by persistently high autoantibody titers, elevated serum immunoglobulins (IgG), cellular infiltration, and beneficial response to corticosteroid therapy.

Serologically, the disease is usually associated with a positive LE cell test and negative hepatitis B antigen. The most pertinent immunologic feature is an elevation in smooth muscle antibodies ($> 1:80$), which persists for many years (21). Patients with viral hepatitis also have a high incidence of SMA but titers are generally low, rarely exceeding $1:80$, and are transient (56).

SMA are found in 70% of CAH sera, however, they have also been detected in up to 46% of patients with primary biliary cirrhosis (31c). Patients with various malignant tumors, infectious mononucleosis, and asthma also demonstrate SMA in their sera. (21, 124, 127). It has been proposed that SMA may be directed against actin, one of the major components of muscle fiber (39).

The IIF technique is the method most often used for SMA detection. Rat stomach cryostat tissue sections are overlayed with diluted suspect sera. FITC-labeled antihuman γ-globulin is added to the system. If SMA are present, they will bind to the muscularis mucosa, resulting in a brilliant apple-green fluorescence. Other suitable substrates are human stomach and monkey or human uterus.

Clearly, a differential diagnosis of chronic active hepatitis cannot be dependent upon the presence or absence of SMA alone. However, the IIF-SMA test, in conjunction with other pertinent laboratory and clinical findings, can be a significant diagnostic aid in differentiating CAH from other liver disease syndromes.

3. Association of Mitochondrial Antibodies with Primary Biliary Cirrhosis

Primary biliary cirrhosis (PBC) is a progressive nonsuppurative liver malady characterized by chronic inflammatory destruction of the small intrahepatic biliary ducts. In the late stages of this disease, the development of portal fibrosis and cirrhosis is not uncommon. PBC is most often found in women between 30 and 60 years of age and is symptomatically characterized by progressive jaundice of unknown etiology.

Serologically, 84–94% of patients with PBC develop high titer circulating mitochondrial autoantibodies (MA) (123). This immunologic abberation is a characteristic feature of the disease and has proved to be a significant diagnostic marker (47, 52).

Again, the IIF technique is the method of choice for the demonstration of mitochondrial antibodies. Unfixed cryostat human or rat kidney sections are most suitable substrates since mitochondrial antigenic determinants are located in the distal tubular epithelium. PBC sera exhibit intense mitochondrial fluorescence at titers above 1:10 (21). Human kidney sections are preferable since nonspecific fluorescence is diminished; however, rat kidney sections are more accessable and give satisfactory results.

MA are not specific for PBC since they are found in 25–30% of patients with CAH and other liver-related disorders (21). The normal population, however, demonstrates a less than 1% incidence of MA (21, 117). Consequently, as in other autoantibody detection systems, positive results should be interpreted with caution and correlated with clinical symptoms and other laboratory data.

B. Immunopathology of the Thyroid Gland

In 1957, Witebsky *et al.* (132a) discussed the phenomenon of autoimmunity in relation to specific cases of chronic thyroiditis. His was one of the early contributions on the subject of autoimmunity. A few years later, Burnett's Forbidden Clone Theory (19a) gave support to Witebsky's Hypothesis. The phenomenon Burnett described involved forbidden clone proliferation, i.e., mutated cells that produced new clones of self-reactive lymphocytes. This mutation resulted in altered self-recognition with subsequent tissue damage.

The fortuitous discovery of the obese strain chickens, (128) also led to a better understanding of autoimmune thyroiditis. This animal model is a specific strain of leghorn chicken, destined to develop spontaneous autoimmune thyroiditis. The animals are characteristically small in size and excessively overweight. Extensive investigation revealed (1) the absence of T3 and T4 proteins, (2) high titers of autoantibodies directed against thyroglobulin (in just 3–4 weeks after hatching), and (3) lymphocytic infiltration with subsequent destruction of the thyroid follicles.

In spite of extensive animal research, human chronic thyroiditis (or Hashimoto's thyroiditis) is still a disease of unknown etiology. It is immunologically mediated and histologically characterized by diffuse lymphocytic infiltration with marked destruction of the normal architecture of the thyroid follicle.

Organ-specific autoantibodies are found in 80% of patients with Hashimoto's thyroiditis (6). There are three distinct thyroid-specific antigen–antibody systems detected by immunofluorescence.

1. Thyroglobulin antibodies—directed against thyroglobulin antigenic sites within the lumen of the thyroid follicle.
2. Microsomal antibodies—directed against the cytoplasmic constituents of epithelial cells lining the follicles.
3. Second colloid antibodies—directed against a second antigen of the acinar colloid, which is localized in some but not all follicles. The clinical relevance and diagnostic usefulness of this autoantibody has not yet been determined, since they are found in both normal patients and in patients with autoimmune thyroiditis (31a).

Thyroid autoantibodies (TA) are detected by several techniques. The tanned red cell hemagglutination method (93b) for thyroglobulin detection is a method of proven reliability. The IIF test is also a valuable technique since all three autoantibody systems can be demonstrated with one substrate. Monkey or human thyroid sections are most often used because they contain all necessary antigenic sites.

Regardless of the method used, TA detection is imperative when a patient presents with evidence of thyroid dysfunction. Negative results for thyroglobulin and microsomal antibodies usually excludes Hashimoto's thyroiditis as a working diagnosis.

Although TA are consistently associated with Hashimoto's thyroiditis, they are also frequently found in Grave's disease, myxedema, rheumatoid arthritis, pernicious anemia, SLE, and thyroid carcinoma (21, 81, 92b).

As previously stated, TA are not pathognomonic for autoimmune thyroiditis, and results must be carefully interpreted.

C. Immunopathology of Skin

1. SLE

The dermatologists of the 1900s had an admittedly incomplete understanding of the concept of autoimmunization. The characteristic SLE dermatologic lesions were thought to be etiologically mediated by the tubuculous bacillus.

Today, IgG antibodies are routinely found in 90% of SLE skin lesions and in 60% of clinically normal SLE skin (120). Histologically, there is marked degeneration of the basal cells. The damage is probably mediated by immune complex deposition in the dermal–epidermal junction (113). IgG is the predominant immunoglobulin involved, however IgM, IgA, and C3 are also frequently demonstrated (28).

A skin biopsy can be an extremely valuable diagnostic tool. Grossman *et al.* (49) have shown that skin biopsies usually reflect nephropathy and may thus obviate the trauma of a kidney biopsy.

2. Pemphigus and Bullous Pemphigoid

Pemphigus is an uncommon autoimmune skin disease, which is characterized by blister formation at the dermoepidermal junction. Patients with active disease demonstrate antiskin autoantibodies and titers correlate with the extent of disease severity (9). The primary immunoglobulin involved is IgG, however IgA and IgM have been detected in some cases (118). IFA tests reveal a characteristic intracullular fluorescence of the prickle cells (9). In bullous pemphigoid, a specific IFA staining of the subepithelial basement zone is demonstrated. As in pemphigus, autoantibody titers correlate with the extent and severity of the disease process.

V. ETIOLOGY OF AUTOIMMUNITY

The etiology of autoimmune disease remains an enigma. Several etiologic hypotheses have been put forth in the last two decades, some have survived whereas others have been supplanted by new ideas.

A. Forbidden Clone Theory

Burnett's theory of autoimmunity(7, 19a) suggests that the immunosurveillance system seeks and destroys antigenically positive (ag+), somatically mutated lymphocytes. These mutants carry antigenic markers and are clearly recognized as foreign. If, however, mutated lymphocytes are lacking antigenic markers (ag−), they will go undetected and proliferate into forbidden clones. These immunocytes will subsequently react with "self" antigenic determinants on target tissues since they are no longer genetically identical.

B. Sequestered Antigen Theory

One of the earliest hypotheses of organ specific-immunity was based on the principle of immunologically induced tolerance during fetal development (7, 81, 92b). This theory assumed that tissues exposed to the lymphoreticular system during embryonic life were "stamped self" and tolerance was induced. Antigens sequestered behind tissue barriers were not recognized as self. Eye lens protein, milk casein, thyroid and testicular tissues were considered hidden antigens. After birth, any mishap such as trauma or infection would lead to the exposure of these formerly sequestered antigens. This state of events would provoke an immune response against the foreign antigens and ultimately result in autoimmunization. The pathogenesis of autoimmune thyroiditis, uveitis, and aspermatogenesis was explained by this proposed mechanism.

Newly developed radioimmunoassay techniques can detect infinitely small amounts of protein in the circulatory system. Investigation of thyroglobulin, for example, has revealed that it is not hidden within the thyroid follicle, but rather equilibrates between the intra- and extracellular fluid around the follicles. (81) Thyroglobulin has the characteristics of other serum proteins and is in contact with the thyroid lymphatics while en route to the circulatory system. Thyroglobulin has been found in the serum of neonates (92a). Consequently, this finding disproves the sequestered antigen theory as the mechanism involved in autoimmune thyroiditis (81).

C. Viral or Neoantigen Theory

The concept of microbial infection as an etiologic agent of autoimmune disease is not new. Recent progress in our understanding of infection has heralded new research in the realm of virally induced autoimmune disease.

The viral hypothesis (25) contends that immunocompetent individuals successfully combat viral insult. In genetically predisposed immunodeficient hosts, however, chronic viral infection may alter "self" antigenic components or the viral coat may eventually contain host cellular constituents. These antigenic abberations result in the formation of a "neoantigen" that is no longer recognized as self. Autoantibodies are produced and may combine with "shedding" neoantigens to form immune complexes or may bind to fixed neoantigens present on infected cell membranes. Whatever the mechanism, immune complex formation seems to lead to the activation of the inflammatory response with the development of autoimmunity.

The scientific basis for this theory is largely dependent on experimental studies involving the NZB/W F1 hybrid mice (11), an animal model destined to develop a syndrome remarkably similar to systemic lupus erythematosus.

VI. MURINE MODEL OF SLE

The fortuitous discovery of the NZB/NZW F1 hybrid murine model (11) led to a more complete understanding of the pathogenesis, treatment, and prognosis of SLE.

Extensive investigation of the NZB/W model showed that after just two months of age, the mice spontaneously developed ANA against double- and single-stranded DNA (112b, 112e). At 4 months, LE cells were demonstrated. This phenomenon was accompanied by complement activation and immune complex deposition in the glomerular basement membrane. Shortly thereafter, the mice developed a rapidly progressive lethal glomerulonephritis and died of renal shutdown by 10–15 months of age (112b, 112e). Another significnat finding was that virgin females developed the most fulminant form of renal disease and died at an even earlier age (19b, 112b, 112e).

Further immunologic investigation of the NZB/W mice provided a foundation for a new working hypothesis that described a genetically predetermined imbalance in T and B cell clones (112c). Young animals normally show a depressed immunologic response and require several weeks to achieve immunologic maturity. NZB/W mice proved to be an exception to that rule. It was noted that 1-week-old NZB/W mice exhibited an antibody response to sheep red blood cells comparable to adults of another strain (89). A selective hyper-responsiveness to synthetic mucleic acids was also found (107). In addition, adult mice were resistant to the induction and maintenance of tolerance when injected with soluble proteins, such as bovine serum albumin (105). Abnormal cell-mediated response was further evidenced by a decreased T cell response to phytomitogens (70) (stimulate T cell proliferation) and impaired tumor rejection (20).

Through these studies, an immunologic premise was established. T cell mediated response was found to be depressed and B cell activity was abnormally hyperactive (112a).

The magnitude of antibody formation is controlled by T suppressor cells (40). Though the mechanism of suppression remains elusive, this subpopulation of T cells seems to be an integral part of tolerance and self–nonself descrimination (15, 112a, 112c). Dauphinee and Talal (29) have demonstrated a T suppressor cell deficinecy in NZB/W mice preceding the onset of autoimmune disease symptoms. The loss of T suppressor cells may be related to a deficiency in thymosin, a thymic hormone necessary for T cell maturation (112d). However, when thymosin was administered to young NZB/W mice, some T cell function was restored but no real beneficial response was observed (41b, 112e). T suppressor cell depletion may also occur as a result of natural thymotoxic antibodies, which are produced by B cells and directed against T cells (77, 102).

In summary, the abnormal immunologic sequence toward the development of autoimmunity in the NZB/W murine model is as follows:

1. There is a decrease in thymic hormone at a very early age.
2. Hormonal deficiency leads to a decline in T suppressor cells and T cell tolerance.
3. At 3–7 months of age, autoantibodies are produced, along with tissue lymphocytic infiltration, immune complex nephritis, and coomb's positive hemolytic anemia.
4. As the animals age (11–13 months), cell-mediated immunity is decreased and lymphoma and monoclonal macroglobulins appear.
5. By the age of 13–14 months, the animals die of progressive lethal glomerulonephritis (112e).

Mellors and Huang (76a) explored the possibility that the immunologic abberations characteristic of NZB/W mice may be caused by a type C virus. They inoculated weanling NZB mice with a filterable agent extracted from NZB lymphoma tissue. The young animals developed several pathologic changes evident in older animals. Electron microscopy revealed the presence of tubular structures consistent with type C viruses.

Other groups of investigators studied the relationship between type C viruses and NZB/W autoimmunity. The following results were reported.

1. Murine leukemias and lymphomas were found to be caused by type C viruses (108).
2. Old NZB/W mice had a high incidence of lymphoma (76b).
3. NZB/W mice are infected with murine leukemia virus from embryo to death (33).

4. The glomerulonephritis developed by this animal model may involve type C virus since this antigen has been found in immune complex deposits (71).

It has been postulated that after host cell infection with type C virus, an enzyme called reverse transcriptase is capable of changing the viral RNA code into DNA. This transcription may then be integrated into the mouse genome, thereby affecting immune responsiveness (108, 114).

Tonietti *et al.* (116) observed that lymphocytic choriomeningitis and polyoma (RNA and DNA viruses, respectively), both intensified autoimmune disease manifestations in NZB/W mice, even though they were dissimilar in viral structure. The authors reported an increase in ANA titers, aggravation of active glomerulonephritis, and increased mortality.

Are these viral particles simply ubiquitous in NZB mice (135) or are they the etiologic agent involved in autoimmunity? The question remains unresolved.

VII. PATHOGENESIS OF HUMAN SLE

Extensive research in the realms of immunopathology, genetics, endocrinology, and virology has lead to a multifactorial concept of SLE pathogenesis. The most prominent etiologic theories are genetic predisposition, endocrinologic factors, immunologic abnormalities at both the cellular and humoral levels, and chronic viral and/or environmental factors.

A. Genetic Predisposition

The major histocompatibility gene complex of man is called HLA. HLA antigens are cell surface glycoproteins involved in cellular interactions and immune responsiveness. They are clincially significant in transplantation rejection, transfusion reactions, and disease susceptibility and resistance.

The association of HLA specificities with certain disease states has been well documented (16). HLA-B27 antigen, a specific gene marker, has been found in 88–90% of caucasian patients with ankylosing spondylitis (133). This finding led investigators to search for specific HLA antigens in SLE patients.

Grumet *et al.* (50) reported a preponderance of two histocompatibility antigens, HL-A8 (33%) and W15 (LND) 40% in SLE patients, compared with a control population of 16 and 10% , respectively. It was proposed that SLE may be associated with an abnormal histocompatibility linked immune response to viral infection and or cellular mutation. Gleland *et al.* (26) also suggested a linkage of an SLE susceptibility factor to the major histocompatibility complex.

The relevance of immunogenetic factors was also reported by Goldberg *et al.* (46). A high incidence of HL-A1 and HL-A8 was found to be associated with severe SLE symptoms such as renal and central nervous system involvement. Currently, a new distinct histocompatibility determinants have been reported in cases of SLE and rheumatoid arthritis (43). Conversely, a study of 65 Danish SLE patients demonstrated no consistent pattern of HLA antigens (61).

A racial predisposition to SLE has also been observed (37). Comparative epidemiological studies revealed that the risk of SLE development was three times greater in black women than in white women. Socioeconomic variables might influence the increased incidence, but a fundamental defect in the immune response seems more likely (103).

Nies *et al.* (82) found HL-A5 in 23 out of 40 black patients compared with 5 out of 120 black controls. Others have studied HLA antigens in black SLE patients. Again, the results were conflicting (13,106).

Another observation that suggests genetic predisposition is the greater concordance for SLE in monozygous twins compared with dizygous twins (14a). In a study performed by Block and Christian(14b) SLE was found in approximately 1–2% of first degree relatives of SLE patients.

The increased incidence of SLE in C2 complement-deficient patients has also been well documented (2, 44, 97, 109). Osterland *et al.* (83) presented an SLE patient with homozygous C2 deficiency manifesting immunologic, dermatologic, renal, and CNS involvement. Familial studies revealed the development of discoid lupus erythematosus in a maternal grand aunt, who was the only other family member with the identical homozygous C2 deficiency. Other family members were studied but no immunologic abberations were detected in two normal and five heterozygous C2 deficient members.

Gewurtz *et al.* (42) also reported a patient with C2 homozygous deficiency and SLE complicated by fulminant lethal nephritis. Investigation of the various components of the complement system and histocompatibility antigens led to the implication of the alternative complement pathway as the mediator of renal damage.

It has been suggested that C2 deficiency may predispose the host to chronic viral infection—thereby setting the stage for immunization against nuclear components with the consequential development of autoimmunity (4).

B. Endocrinology

Endocrine factors represent yet another mechanism involved in the pathogenesis of SLE. Investigators of the NZB/W model raised the question—why does SLE develop with more severity and at an earlier age in the NZB/W female? Talal *et al.* (112e) studied the sequential development of IgM and IgG antibodies to RNA and DNA. The data suggested that the thymus, spleen, and gonads exerted major regulatory influences. They also found that androgen treatment exerted a protective effect in NZB/W mice. Immune complex nephritis was reduced and female survival was prolonged.

Prepubertal castration of male NZB/W mice at 2 weeks of age resulted in an acceleration of autoantibodies directed against DNA and increased disease-associated mortality (112e). In addition, it was found that estrogen therapy accelerated female mortality whereas androgen treatment prolonged the survival rate (96). Androgen administration to both male and female mice lowered anti-DNA antibody titers and decreased immune complex associated nephritis (112e). The data obtained from these studies suggests that the expression of autoimmunity in NZB/W mice may be modulated by sex hormones.

Unfortunately, endocrine manipulation in humans has not been as successful. When female SLE patients were treated with massive doses of testosterone, no therapeutic effect was observed. In addition, maintenance androgen therapy without corticosteroid treatment did not maintain clinical remission (32a). Results are still conflicting for in 1975 Yocum *et al.* (134) reported a case of monozygous twins discordant for SLE. Comparison studies were performed on autoantibody production, viral antibody titers, γ-globulin, and light chain metabolism. The most striking finding was that the healthy twin had undergone bilateral oophorectomy at a young age.

C. Immunologic Abnormalities

There is convincing evidence that patients with active SLE demonstrate a general hyporeactivity or impaired cell-mediated response (53b, 95). Horowitz and Cousar (57) compared the relationship between impaired cellular immunity, humoral suppression of lymphocyte function, and the severity of SLE. Eighteen untreated SLE patients were divided into two groups based on severe or mild active disease. Cell-mediated response was measured by delayed hypersensitivity skin test antigens and lymphocytic reactivity was assessed by response to mitogen stimulation. The patients with severe active SLE were nonresponsive to skin test antigens and demonstrated impaired cell-mediated immunity whereas most patients with mild active disease showed intact cell-mediated response. Normal lymphocyte function was demonstrated *in vitro*, since lymphocytes from both groups of patients responded normally to phytohemagglutination (PHA) stimulation.

Of special interest, was the discovery of an immunosuppressive IgG (termed lymphocyte regulatory globulin) in the serum of SLE patients with severe active disease. The degree of lymphocytic suppression to PHA stimulation correlated with impaired cell-mediated response and disease severity. Data from other laboratories supported this finding (126, 129). Unfortunately lymphocyte regulatory globulin does not appear to be specific for SLE since similar immunologic abnormalities were found in patients with primary intracranial tumors (17).

Nevertheless, data from these studies support the hypothesis put forth by investigators of the NZB/W model—an immunologic imbalance between B and T cell clones characterized by an enhanced or hyperactive humoral response and a hypoactive or depressed cell-mediated response. This immunologic abberation may be mediated by a lack of T suppressor cells and or a thymic hormone deficiency.

The intact immunosurveillance system operates by many different T- and B-cell subpopulations and is controlled by delicate feedback mechanisms. After antigenic stimulation and lymphocytic proliferation at both cellular and humoral levels, the immune response must be "shut-off" or suppressed. Indeed, if antibody-responding lymphocytes continued to proliferate without control, antibody titers would continually increase and our serum would soon take on the consistency of syrup—a condition incompatible with life. An example of this disorder is multiple myeloma, a neoplastic disease accompanied by high globulin blood levels and immunologically characterized by uncontrolled lymphocytic proliferation.

In autoimmune disease, overproduction of autoantibody by B cell clones seems to be caused by a decrease in suppressor T cells. This lymphopenia may be due to lymphocytotoxic antibodies, which are frequently found in the serum of SLE patients (79) and NZB/W mice (102). These antibodies are capable of destroying T lymphocytes and interfering with the functional activity of T suppressor cells. T suppressor cell depletion may also be caused by a premature loss of thymic hormone (3, 67).

D. Viral Factors

The part that viruses play in the etiology of SLE still remains hypothetical. As with other diseases of unknown etiology the viral and or microbial infection hypothesis still remains attractive.

Viral evidence accumulated from the NZB/W model has focused attention on the role of type C viruses in the pathogenesis of human SLE. Fresco (38) recognized tubular myxoviruslike structures in glomerular deposits from a case of lupus nephritis.

Gyorkey et al. (51) described similar inclusion particles in SLE glomerular epithelium. In most cases, the inclusion particles resembled at least superficially the nucleocapsids of the paramyxoviruses. These RNA viruses include many common human pathogens such as mumps, measles, parainfluenzae, and various respiratory viruses.

Evidence accumulated from clinical case histories suggests that a causative agent may be transplacentally transmitted from mother to fetus (18). Studies with the NZB/W model support this hypothesis (71).

Although many groups of investigators support the viral hypothesis, considerable negative evidence has also been presented. For example, later studies have shown that electron microscopic inclusion particles found in SLE glomerular epithelium are not consistent with any known virus (99). Imamura et al. (58) found type C viruslike particles in normal as well as SLE placentas. The significance of these viruslike inclusion particles still remains debatable. Perhaps, they are merely cellular debris (87a).

In addition, repeated attempts at type C viral isolation from SLE tissue were negative (73, 87b). Other sophisticated viral detection methods were also negative (23).

VIII. CONCLUSION

The data presented is controversial, to say the least, and does not provide adequate evidence for any one theory of pathogenesis. Conceivably, all factors are involved and interrelated. There may well turn out to be further research complexities encountered since the pathologic mechanism of autoimmunity is a dynamic system. The etiology may still remain an enigma, however, one must not forget the turbulent history involved in the *acceptance* of autoimmunity as a disease phenomenon. Just 20 years ago, Witebsky fought for the recognition of a disease process mediated by an abnormal immune system. At that time well-respected colleagues refused to believe in "such a thing as an autoantibody" (132b). Two decades later the theory of autoimmunization is an accepted fact. This evolution of thought illustrates the path by which progress is achieved in science.

REFERENCES

1. Aarden, L. A., de Groot, E. R., and Feltkamp, T. E. W. (1975). *Ann. N.Y. Acad. Sci.* **254,** 505–515.
2. Angello, V., DeBracco, M. M. E., and Kunkel, H. G. (1972). *J. Immunol.* **108,** 837–840.
3. Bach, J. F., Dardenne, M., and Solomon, J. C. (1973). *Clin. Exp. Immunol.* **14,** 247–256.
4. Bardana, E. J., Jr., and Pirofsky, B. (1975). *West. J. Med.* **122,** 130–144.
5. Barret, J. T. (1974). "Textbook of Immunology" p. 14, 306–309, 99–129. C. V. Mosby Company, St. Louis, Missouri.
6. Beall, G. N., and Solomon, D. H. (1973). *Postgrad. Med.* **54,** 181.
7. Bellanti, J. A. (1971). *In* "Immunology" (Rosalie E. Green, ed.), pp. 341–431. Saunders, Philadelphia, Pennsylvania.
8. Bendixen, G. (1971). *In* "Clinical Hypersensitivity Disorders." I. (Newton Kugelmass, ed.) pp. 27–30. Thomas, Springfield, Illinois.
9. Beutner, E. H., Jordan, R. E., and Chorzelski, T. P. (1968). *J. Invest. Dermatol.* **51,** 63–80.
10. Bickel, Y. B., Barnett, E. V., and Pearson, C. M. (1968). *Clin. Exp. Immunol.* **3,** 641–656.
11. Bielschowsky, M., Helyer, B. J., and Howie, J. B. (1959). *Proc. Univ. Otago Med. Sch.* **37,** 9–11.
12. BioScience Laboratories (1976). "New Test Summaries from BioScience Laboratories," pamphlet, pp. 1–2. BioScience Enterprises Pub., Los Angeles, California.
13. Bitter, T., Mottironi, W. D., and Terasaki, P. I. (1972). *N. Engl. J. Med.* **286,** 435–436.
14a. Block, S. R., Winfield, J. B., Lockshin, M. D., D'Angelo, W. A., and Christian, C. L. (1975). *Am. J. Med.* **59,** 533–552.
14b. Block, S. R., and Christian, C. L. (1975). *Am. J. Med.* **59,** 453–456.
15. Borel, Y. (1976). *Transplant. Rev.* **31,** 3–22.
16. Brewerton, D. A. (1976). *Arthritis Rheum.* **19,** 656.
17. Brooks, W. H., Netsky, M. G., Normansell, D. E. and Horowitz, D. A. (1972). *J. Exp. Med.* **136,** 1631–1647.
18. Brustein, D., Rodriguez, J. M., Minkin, W., and Rabhan, N. B. (1977). *JAMA* **238,** 2294–2296.
19a. Burnett, F. M. (1959). *Brit. Med. J.* **2,** 720–725.
19b. Burnett, F. M., and Holmes, M. C. (1965). *Aust. Ann. Med.* **14,** 185.
20. Cantor, H., Asofsky, R., and Talal, N. (1970). *J. Exp. Med.* **131,** 223–234.
21. Cavallaro, J. J., Palmer, D. F., and Bigazzi, P. E., (1976) "Immunofluorescence Detection of Autoimmune Diseases" pp. 1, 7, 8, 24, 86, 87. U.S. Department of Health Education and Welfare Public Health Service, Center for Disease Control, Atlanta, Ga.
22. Chandor, S. B. (1976). *In* "Laboratory Tests in the Diagnosis of Autoimmune Disorders" R. M. (R. M. Nakamura and S. Deodhar, eds.), p. 139. Amer. Soc. Clin. Pathol., Chicago, Illinois.
23. Charman, H. P., and Phillips, P. E. (1977). *Arthritis Rheum.* **20,** 110. (Abst.)
24. Chubick, A., Sontheimer, R. D., Gilliam, J. N., and Ziff, M. (1978). *Ann. Int. Med.* **89,** 186–192.
25. Christian, C. L., and Phillips, P. E. (1973). *Am. J. Med. 54,* 611–620.
26. Cleland, L. G., Bell, D. A., Martin, W., and Saurino, B. C. (1978). *Arthritis Rheum.* **21,** 183–191.
27a. Coons, A. H., and Kaplan, M. H. (1950). *J. Exp. Med.* **91,** 1–13.

27b. Coons, A. H. (1951). *Fed. Proc.* **10**, 558–559.

28. Cormane, R. H. *et al.* (1966). *Clin. Exp. Immunol.* **1**, 207–212. Ballieux, R. E., Kalsbeek, G. L. and Hymans, W.

29. Dauphinee, M. J., and TaLal, N. (1973). *Proc. Natl. Acad. Sci. U.S.A.* Part II, **70**, 3769–3773.

30. Davies, P., and Allison, A. C. (1976). *In* "Immunobiology of the Macrophage" (D. S. Nelson, ed.), pp. 428–457. Academic Press, New York.

31a. Doniach, D., and Roitt, I. M. (1968). *In* "Clinical Aspects of Immunology" (P. G. H. Gell and R. R. A. Coombs, eds.), pp. 933–958 Blackwell Scientific Publications, Oxford.

31b. Doniach, D. (1972). *Prog. Clin. Immunol.* **1**, 45–70.

31c. Doniach, D., and Walker, G. (1972). *In* "Progress in Liver Disease" (H. Popper and F. Schaffner, eds.), p. 381. Grune and Stratton, New York.

32a. Dubois, E. L., Commons, R. R., Starr, P., Stein, C. S., Jr., and Morrison, R. (1952). *JAMA* **149**, 995–1002.

32b. Dubois, E. L. (1971). *Semin. Arthritis Rheum.* **1**, 97–102.

32c. Dubois, E. L., ed. (1974). *In* "Lupus Erythematosus," pp. 1, 10, 487–524. Univ. of Southern California Press, Los Angeles, California.

32d. Dubois, E. L. (1975). *J. Rheum.* **2**, 204–214.

33. East, J., Prosser, P. R., Holborow, E. J., and Jaquet, H. (1967). *Lancet* **1**, 755.

34. Edelman, G. M. (1973). *Science* **180**, 830–840. (Nobel Lecture.)

35a. Ehrlick, P., and Margenroth, J. (1900). *Klin. Wochenschr.* **37**, 453.

35b. Ehrlick, P. (1906). *Proc. Roy. Soc. London, Ser. B* **66**, 424.

36. Farr, R. D. (1958). *J. Infect. Dis.* **103**, 239.

37. Fessel, W. J. (1974). *Arch. Intern. Med.* **134**, 1027–35.

38. Fresco, R. (1968). *Fed. Proc.* **27**, 246–51.

39. Gabbiani, G., Ryan, G. B., Lamlin, J. P., Vassalli, P., Majno, G., Bouvier, C. Cruchaud, A., and Lucher E. (1973). *Am. J. Pathol.* **72**, 473–488.

40. Gershon, R. K. (1974). *In* "Contemporary Topics in Immunolobiology" (M. D. Cooper and N. L. Warner, eds.), pp. 1–40. Plenum, New York.

41a. Gershwin, M. E., and Steinberg, A. D. (1974). *Arthritis Rheum.* **17**, 947–954.

41b. Gershwin, M. E., Steinberg, A. D., Ahmed, A. Derkay, C. (1976). *Arthritis Rheum.* **19**, 862–866.

42. Gerwurtz, A., Lent, T. F., Roberts, J. L., Leitz, H., and Gewurtz, H. (1978). *Arthritis Rheum.* **21**, 28–36.

43. Gibofsky, A., Winchester, R., Hansen, J., Patarroyo, M., Dupont, B., Paget, S., Lahita, R., Halper, J. Fotino, M., Yunis, E., and Kunkel, H. G. (1978). *Arthritis Rheum. Suppl.* **21**, S134–138.

44. Glass, D., Raum, D., Gibson, D., Stillman, J. S., and Schur, P. H. (1976). *J. Clin. Invest.* **58**, 853–861.

45. Goel, K. M., Shanks, R. A., Shaley, K., Mason, M., and MacSween, R. N. M. (1975). *Arch. Dis. Child.* **50**, 419.

46. Goldberg, M. A., Arnett, F. C., Beas, W. B., and Shulman, L. E. (1973). *Arthritis Rheum.* **16**, 546–547.

47. Goudie, R. B., MacSween, R. N. M., and Goldberg, D. M. (1966). *J. Clin. Pathol.* **19**, 527–538.

48. Greaves, M. F., Owen, J. J. T., and Raff, M. C. (1973). "T and B Lymphocytes." Amer. Elsevier, New York.

49. Grossman, J., Callerame, M. L., and Condemi, J. J. (1974). *Ann. Intern. Med.* **80**, 496–499.

50. Grumet, F. C., Coukell, A., Bodmer, J. G., Bodmer, W. F., and McDevitt, H. O. (1971). *N. Engl. J. Med.* **285**, 193–196.
51. Gyorkey, F., Sinkovics, J. G., Min, K. W., and Gyorkey, P. (1972). *Am. J. Med.* **53**, 148–158.
52. Hadziyannis, S., Scheuer, P. J., Feizi, T., Naccaratto, R., Doniach, D., and Sherlock, S. (1970). *J. Clin. Pathol.* **23**, 95–8.
53a. Hahn, B. H., Sharp, G. C., Irvin, W. S., Kantor, O. S. Gardner, C. A., Bagby, M. K., Perry, H. M., and Osterland, C. K. (1972). *Ann. Intern. Med.* **76**, 365–374.
53a. Hahn, B. H., Bagby, M. K., and Osterland, C. K. (1973). *Am. J. Med.* **55**, 25–31.
54. Hargraves, M. M., Richmond, H., and Morton, R. (1948). *Mayo Clin. Proc.* **23**, 25–28.
55. Hobart, M. J., McConnel, I. and Valdimarsson, H., (1975). *In* "The Immune System: A Course on the Molecular and Cellular Basis of Immunity" (M. J. Hobart, and I. McConnel, eds.), pp. 3, 9, 98, 181. Blackwell, Oxford.
56. Holborow, E. J. (1972). *Proc. Roy. Soc. Med.* **65**, 481–4.
57. Horowitz, D. A., and Cousar, J. B. (1975). *Am. J. Med.* **58**, 829–835.
58. Imamura, M., Phillips, P. E., and Mellors, R. C. (1976). *Am. J. Pathol.* **83**, 383–394.
59. Ishizaka, K., and Ishzaka T. (1971). *Clin. Allergy* **1**, 9–24.
60. Johnson, G. D., Holborow, E. J., and Glynn, L. E. (1965). *Lancet* **2**, 878–90.
61. Kissmeyer-Nielsen F., Kjerbye, K., Andersen, E. and Halberg, P. (1975). *Transplant. Rev.* **22**, 164–167.
62. Klatskin, G., and Kantor, F. S. (1972). *Ann. Intern. Med.* **77**, 533–41.
63a. Koffler, D., Schur, P. H., and Kunkel, H. G. (1967). *J. Exp. Med.* **126**, 607–624.
63b. Koffler, D., Agnello, V., Thoburn, R., and Kunkel, H. G. (1971). *J. Exp. Med. Suppl.* **134**, 169S–179S.
63c. Koffler, D., Agnello, V., and Kunkel, H. G. (1974). *Am. J. Pathol.* **74**, 109–24.
64. Kredich, N. M., Skyler, J. S., and Foote, L. J. (1973). *Arch. Intern. Med.* **131**, 639–644.
65. Krishnan, C., and Kaplan, M. H. (1967). *J. Clin. Invest.* **46**, 569–579.
66. Kunkel, H. G., and Williams, R. C. (1964). *Annu. Rev. Med.* **15**, 37–52.
67. Kysela, S., and Steinberg, A. D. (1973). *Clin. Immunol. Immunopathol.* **2**, 133–136.
68. Lee, S. L., and Chase, P. H. (1975). *Semin. Arthritis Rheum.* **5**, 83–103.
69. Lerner, R. A., and Dixon, F. J. (1966). *J. Exp. Med.* **124**, 431–442.
70. Leventhal, B. G., and Talal, N. (1970). *J. Immunol.* **104**, 918–923.
71. Levy, J. A. (1974). *Am. J. Clin. Pathol.* **62**, 258–280.
72. Lightfoot, R. W., Redecha, P. B., Leve, S., and Anos, N. (1975). *Scand. J. Rheumatol. Suppl.* **11**, 52–58.
73. Markenson, J. A., Phillips, P. E., Brinkmann, J. P., Snyder, H. W., and Christian, C. L. (1977). *Clin. Res.* **25**, 485.
74. Marx, J. L. (1975). *Science* **182**, 245–247.
75. Matre, R., Helgeland, S. M., and Tonder, O. (1974). *J. Immunol. Methods* **5**, 345.
76a. Mellors, R. C., and Huang, C. Y. (1966). *J. Exp. Med.* **124**, 1031–1038.
76b. Mellors, R. C. (1966). *Int. Rev. Exp. Pathol.* **5**, 217–221.
77. Messner, R. P., and DeHoratius, R. J. (1978). *Arthritis Rheum. Suppl.* **21**, S167–S170.
78. Metchnikoff, E. (1905). "Immunity in Infectious Diseases." Cambridge Univ. Press, London and New York.
79. Mittal, K. K., Rosen, R. D.,and Sharp, J. T. (1970). *Nature (London)* **225**, 1255–1256.
80a. Müller-Eberhard, H. J., and Calcott, M. A. (1966). *Immunochemistry* **3**, 500.
80b. Müller-Eberhard, H. J. (1975). *Annu. Rev. Biochem.* **44**, 697–724.
81. Kakamaura, R. M., Doedhar, S. and Tucker, E. S. (1976). *In* "Laboratory Tests in the

Diagnosis of Autoimmune Disorders" (R. M. Nakamura and S. Deodhar, eds.), pp. 6, 57, 103, 120, 162. Amer. Soc. of Clin. Pathol., Chicago, Illinois.

82. Nies, K. M., Brown, J. C., Dubois, E. L., Quismoreo, F. B., Friou, G. J., and Teraski, P. I. (1974). *Arthritis Rheum.* **17,** 397–402.

83. Osterland, C. K., Espinoza, L., Parker, L. P., and Schur, P. H. (1975). *Ann. Intern. Med.* **82,** 323–328.

84. Parker, M. D., (1973). *J. Lab. Clin. Med.* **82,** 769–775.

85a. Paronetto, F., and Popper, H. (1969). *In* "Textbook of Immunopathology" (P. A. Meischer and H. J. Müller-Eberhard, eds.), Vol. II, pp. 562–583. Grune and Stratton, New York.

85b. Paronetto, F. (1970). *In* "Progress in Liver Disease" (H. Popper, ed.), Vol. 3, p. 299. Grune and Stratton, New York.

86. Peter, J. B. (1978). *Diagn. Med.* **1,** 67–80.

87a. Phillips, P. E. (1975). *Clin. Rheum. Dis.* **1,** 505–518.

87b. Phillips, P. E., Hargrave, R., Steward, E., and Sarkar, N. H. (1976). *Ann. Rheum, Dis.* **35,** 422–428.

88. Pike, R. M., Sulkin, S. E., and Coggeshall, H. C. (1949). *J. Immunol.* **63,** 447–463.

89. Playfair, J. H. L. (1968). *Immunology* **15,** 35–50.

90. Porter, R. R. (1973). *In* "Defence and Recognition" (H. L. Kornberg, D. C. Phillips, and R. R. Porter, eds.), pp. 159–197. MTP (International Review of Science) and Butterworth, London.

91. Raff, M. D. (1973). *Nature (London)* **242,** 19.

92a. Roitt, I. M., and Torrigiani, G. (1967). *Endocrinology* **81,** 421–429.

92b. Roitt, I. (1977). "Essential Immunology" pp. 36–38, 40, 161, 272, 276. Blackwell, Oxford.

93a. Rose, H. M., Ragan, C., Pearce, E., and Lipman, O. M. (1948). *Proc. Soc. Exp. Biol. Med.* **68,** 1–6.

93b. Rose, N. R., Bigazzi, P., Bartholomew, W., Wicher, K., Gorznyski, E., and Abeyounis, C. (1973). *In* "Methods in Immunodiagnosis" (N. R. Rose and P. E. Bigazzi, eds.), pp. 51–56. Wiley, New York.

94. Rosenbaum, J. T., and Duryer, J. M. (1977). *Cancer (Philadelphia)* **39,** 11–20.

95. Rosenthal, C. J., and Franklin, E. C. (1973). *Arthritis Rheum.* **16,** 565.

96. Roubinian, J. R., Papoian, R., and Talal, N. (1977). *J. Clin. Invest.* **59,** 1066–1070.

97. Rynes, R. I., Urizar, R. E., and Pickering, R. J. (1977). *Am. J. Med.* **63,** 279–288.

98. Sanders, D. Y., Huntley, C. C., and Sharp, G. C. (1973). *J. Pediat.* **83,** 642–645.

99. Schaff, Z., Barry, D. W., and Grimley, P. M. (1973). *Lab. Invest.* **29,** 577–586.

100. Schur, P. H., and Sandson, J. (1968). *N. Engl. J. Med.* **278,** 533.

101a. Sharp, G. C., Irvin, W. S., Tan, E. M., Gould, R. G., and Holman, H. R. (1972). *Am. J. Med.* **52,** 148–159.

101b. Sharp, G. C. (1974). *Bull. Rheum. Dis.* **25,** 828–831.

101c. Sharp, G. C. (1975). *Clin. Rheum. Dis.* **1,** 561.

102. Shirai, T., and Mellors, R. C. (1971). *Proc. Natl. Acad. Sci. U.S.A.* **68,** 1412–1415.

103. Siegel, M., and Lee, S. L. (1973). *Semin. Arthritis.* **3,** 1–54.

104a. Singer, J. M., and Plotz, C. M. (1956). *Am. J. Med.* **21,** 888–892.

104b. Singer, J. M. (1974). *Bull. Rheum. Dis.* **24,** 762–768.

105. Staples, P. J., Steinberg, A. D., and Talal, N. (1970). *J. Exp. Med.* **131,** 123–28.

106. Stastny, P. (1972). *Arthritis Rheum.* **15,** 455–456.

107. Steinberg, A. D., Baron, S. H., Talal, N. (1969). *Pro. Natl. Acad. Sci. U.S.A.* **63,** 1102–1107.

108. Stephenson, J. R., and Aaronson, S. A. (1972). *Proc. Natl. Acad. Sci.* U.S.A. **69,** 2798.
109. Stern, R., Fu, S. M., Fotini, M., Angello, V., and Kunkel, H. (1976). *Arthritis Rheum.* **19,** 517–522.
110. Stingl, G., Meingassner, J. G., Sweety, P., and Knapp, W. (1976). *Clin. Immunol. Immunopath.* **6,** 131–140.
111. Suyehira, L. A., and Gewurtz, H. (1977). *Lab. Med.* **8,** 29–34.
112a. Talal, N. (1970). *Arthritis Rheum.* **13,** 887.
112b. Talal, N., and Steinberg, A. D. (1974). *Curr. Top. Microbiol. Immunol.* **64,** 79–103.
112c. Talal, N. (1975). *West. J. Med.* **2,** 156–157.
112d. Talal, N., Dauphinee, M. J., Pillarisetty, R., and Goldblum, R. (1975). *Ann. N.Y. Acad. Sci.* **249,** 438–450.
112e. Talal, N. (1978). *Arthritis Rheum. Suppl.* **21,** S58–S63.
113. Tan, E. M., and Kunkel, H. G. (1966). *Arthritis Rheum.* **9,** 37–46.
114. Temin, H. M., and Mizutani, S. (1970). *Nature (London)* **226,** 1211.
115. Tomassi, T. B., and Bienenstock, J. (1968). *Adv. Immunol.* **9,** 1–96.
116. Tonietti, G., Oldstone, M. B. A., and Dixon, F. J. (1970). *J. Exp. Med.* **132,** 89–109.
117. Tourville, D. R. T. (1977). "Clinical Relevance of Autoantibodies" pp. 2–5. Zeus Scientific Publishers, Raritan, N. J.
118. Triftshauser, C., and Beutner, E. H. (1969). *Fed. Proc.* **28,** 770.
119. Tucker, E. S. (1976). *In* "Laboratory Tests in the Diagnosis of Autoimmune Disorders" (R. M. Nakamaura and S. Deodhar, eds.), p. 162. Amer. Soc. of Clin. Pathol., Chicago, Illinois.
120. Tuffanelli, D. L., Kay, D., and Fukurjama, K. (1969). *Arch. Dermatol.* **99,** 652–662.
121. Unanue, E. R., and Dixon, F. S. (1967). *Adv. Immunol.* **6,** 1–7.
122. Waaler, E. (1940). *Acta Pathol. Microbiol. Scand.* **17,** 172–188.
123. Walker, J. G., Doniach, D., Roitt, I. M., and Sherlock, S. (1965). *Lancet* **1,** 827.
124. Warwick, M. T., and Haslam, P. (1970). *Clin. Exp. Immunol.* **7,** 31.
125. Weitzman, R. J., and Walker, S. E. (1976). *Lab. Med.* **7,** 6–10.
126. Wernet, P., and Kunkel, H. G. (1973). *J. Exp. Med.* **138,** 1021.
127. Whitehouse, J. M. A., and Holborow, E. J. (1971). *Br. Med. J.* **4,** 511.
128. Wick, G., Sundick, R. S., and Albini, B. (1974). *Clin. Immunol. Immunopath.* **3,** 272–300.
129. Williams, R. C., Lies, R. B., and Messner, R. P. (1973). *Arthritis Rheum.* **16,** 597.
130. Winchester, R. J. (1975). *Ann. N.Y. Acad. Sci.* **256,** 73–81.
131. Winfield, J. B., Faiferman, I. and Koffler, D. (1977). *J. Clin. Invest.* **59,** 90.
132a. Witebsky, E., Rose, N. R., Terplan, K., Paine, J. R., and Egan, R. W. (1957). *JAMA* **164,** 1439–1447.
132b. Witebsky, E. (1965). *Ann. N.Y. Acad. Sci.* **124,** 978.
133. Woodrow, J. C. (1977). *Semin. Arthritis Rheum.* **6,** 257–76.
134. Yocum, W. M., Grossman, J., Waterhouse, C., Abraham, G. N., Nay, A. G., and Condemi, J. J. (1975). *Arthritis Rheum.* **18,** 193–199.
135. Yoshiki, T., Mellors, R. C., Strand, M., and August, J. T. (1974). *J. Exp. Med.* **140,** 1011.

7

Specific Proteins in Plasma, Cerebrospinal Fluid, Urine, and Other Biological Fluids

LAWRENCE M. KILLINGSWORTH AND CAROL E. KILLINGSWORTH

CLINICAL BIOCHEMISTRY
Contemporary Theories and Techniques, Vol. 1

I. PLASMA PROTEIN PROFILES

A. Overview of Plasma Proteins

The use of plasma protein data to aid in the diagnosis of disease and provide supportive pathophysiological information has increased markedly over the past decade. The most common form of overall protein testing is electrophoresis on either cellulose acetate or agarose gel as a support medium, but specific quantitation of individual proteins as "protein profiles" has also gained acceptance. The development of mechanized equipment for immunochemical analysis has been a contributing factor in the emergence of the specific protein profile as a routine laboratory test (Killingsworth, 1976).

Of the more than 100 plasma proteins that have been characterized biochemically, relatively few have well-documented clinical significance. These are, for the most part, the higher concentration proteins which are within the detection limits of current analytical techniques. Electrophoretic fractionation of serum, as shown in Fig. 1, results in a pattern which is dominated by 13 proteins, but these are not separated into distinct bands, and the interpretive return from this type of study is limited (Laurell, 1972a,b; Kawai, 1973; Sun et al., 1978). Quantitative immunochemical techniques have allowed for a closer inspection of individual plasma protein components with a resultant increase in useful information (Ritchie, 1974a,b; Bouige et al., 1973). A synthetic approach, in which specific protein results and qualitative electrophoretic data are combined with pertinent findings from clinical examination of the patient, has proved to be an effective means of maximizing the clinical value of protein assays (Laurell, 1972b, 1973; Alper, 1974; Killingsworth, 1976, 1978). Profile studies have led to an increased understanding of protein physiology in healthy individuals and helped characterize the complex relationships of proteins in basic pathological processes.

This section will present a summary of plasma protein profiles observed in health and in various disease categories. Results on normal individuals will cover age- and sex-related variations and day-to-day biologic variations. Discussion of patterns frequently observed in disease states will include the inflammatory process, rheumatic diseases, liver diseases, protein-losing disorders, plasma cell dyscrasias, pregnancy and genetic protein deficiencies. A section on management of protein data will discuss interpretive reporting with emphasis on graphical data presentation and pattern recognition.

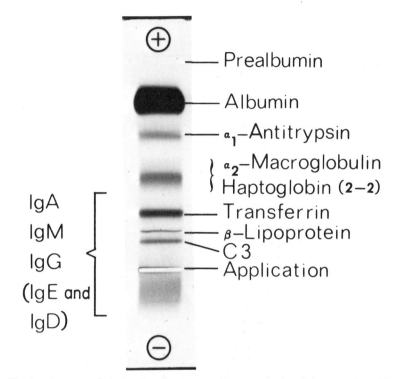

Fig. 1. Agarose gel electrophoretic pattern of serum proteins. Other proteins with relatively high concentrations include α-lipoprotein, α_1-acid glycoprotein, α_1-antichymotrypsin, ceruloplasmin, hemopexin, C4, C1-esterase inhibitor, and fibrinogen (in plasma). (From Killingsworth, L. M. (1979). Plasma protein patterns in health and disease. *Crit. Rev. Clin. Lab. Sci.* **11**, 1–30. Reproduced by permission of the copyright owner.)

B. Plasma Protein Patterns in Health

1. Variations with Age and Sex

a. Cord Blood Pattern. Gitlin and Gitlin (1975a) have published an extensive report on fetal and neonatal protein synthesis. Their most dramatic findings, when expressed as a ratio of the neonatal concentration to the adult concentration, is the α_1-fetoprotein. α_2-Macroglobulin and α_1-antitrypsin concentrations were also found to be greater than mean adult levels. Essentially normal adult quantities of albumin, fibrinogen, IgG, Cl esterase inhibitor, and Gc globulin were observed, with other proteins showing slight to marked decreases. The results of Ganrot (1972) agree closely with those of Gitlin and Gitlin except that slight decreases were

TABLE I[a,b]

Plasma Protein Pattern at Birth

Prealbumin	↓		
Albumin	N or ↓		
α-Lipoprotein	↓		
α$_1$-Acid glycoprotein	↓ ↓		
α$_1$-Antitrypsin	↑ or ↓		
α$_2$-Macroglobulin	↑ ↑		
Ceruloplasmin	↓ ↓		
Haptaglobin	↓ ↓ ↓		
Hemopexin	↓ ↓		
Gc-globulin	N		
Transferrin	↓		
β-Lipoprotein	↓ ↓		
Complement C3	↓		
Complement C4	↓		
Fibrinogen	N		
IgG	N		
IgA	↓ ↓ ↓		
IgM	↓ ↓		
Cl esterase inhibitor	N		
Plasminogen	↓		
α-Fetoprotein	↑ ↑ ↑ ↑		

[a] From Killingsworth, L. M. (1979). Plasma protein patterns in health and disease. *Crit. Rev. Clin. Lab. Sci.* **11,** 1–30. Reproduced by permission of the copyright owner.

[b] Concentrations expressed relative to mean adult levels.

noted in α$_1$-antitrypsin and IgG. Two groups assayed immunoglobulins in normal children, and their results indicated adult levels of IgG with decreases in IgM and marked decreases in IgA at birth (Buckley *et al.*, 1968; Cejka *et al.*, 1974). These studies agree well with conclusions reached by Gitlin and Gitlin (1975a). Complement components C3 and C4 were assessed by Norman *et al.* (1975). Results for C3 were in agreement with two other groups of investigators (Ganrot, 1972; Gitlin and Gitlin, 1975a). The results of all studies are summarized in Table I with greatest weight given to those trends on which several groups agree.

b. Protein Levels throughout Life. Lyngbye and Krøll (1971) evaluated protein variations in a healthy population from ages of 8 to 95 years. No significant age-related variations were seen with prealbumin, ceruloplasmin, α_2-HS globulin, and IgM. Only a slight increase in the male before the age of 30 years was seen in plasminogen. Albumin concentration was constant until the age of 50 years, after which it tended to decrease. α_1-Acid glycoprotein levels tended to increase until 30 years in the male and after 40 years in the female. Values for α_1-lipoprotein and α_1-antitrypsin increased slightly until age 40 years. Haptoglobin showed increasing values with age. A pronounced decrease was seen in α_2-macroglobulin to about age 40 years with increases in older age. Transferrin values decreased until age 40 years in males. Young females exhibited an increase in transferrin, followed by a decrease after age 30 years. Complement C3 showed increasing levels with age in males, with decreasing levels to about age 30 years in females, followed by increases. IgA levels increased throughout life, but the increase tended to diminish at about age 35 years. IgG values decreased slightly until about 50 years of age and increased thereafter. The major sex-related differences were higher levels of ceruloplasmin and transferrin in females during the childbearing years and higher levels of α_2-macroglobulin and IgM in adult females.

Weeke and Krasilnikoff (1971) studied serum proteins in a normal population ranging in age from 1 to 93 years and developed a polynomial expression to describe the concentration changes with age. Their findings indicated prealbumin, lipoproteins, and immunoglobulins increase during early childhood whereas ceruloplasmin and α_2-macroglobulin decrease. Albumin and transferrin were seen to decrease in old age whereas IgG and α_2-macroglobulin increased. These same investigators compared values for proteins in children with those in adults (Weeke and Krasilnikoff, 1972). The children showed significantly lower mean concentration of prealbumin, α_1-lipoprotein, α_1-antitrypsin, α_1-antichymotrypsin, Gc globulin, haptoglobin, hemopexin, β-lipoprotein, IgG, IgA, and IgM. Higher mean concentrations in children were observed with ceruloplasmin and α_2-macroglobulin.

Dramatic changes of immunoglobulin levels in early childhood are well known (Buckley *et al.*, 1968; Alford, 1971; Cejka *et al.*, 1974). There is general agreement as to the levels of all three immunoglobulins at birth. Immunoglobulin G reaches a minimum at about 3 months, as the maternal protein is catabolized, and gradually reaches adult levels at about 7–10 years. Immunoglobulin A concentration steadily increased to adult levels at 12–16 years. There is little agreement concerning immunoglobulin M synthesis. Whereas Buckley and co-workers (1968) found IgM levels to remain below 80% of adult levels until age 14 years, Cejka *et al.* (1974) showed IgM at 83% of adult levels at the 3- to 6-year interval and Alford

(1971) reported attainment of adult levels at 1 year of age. This discrepancy could result from the small populations investigated in each age-group.

A study of serum complement profiles in infants and children (Norman et al., 1975) showed that both C3 and C4 concentrations increased in childhood, reaching about 90% of adult levels by 2 years of age. Essentially adult concentrations are attained by 6 years of age.

2. Individual Variations

Two groups (Statland et al., 1976; Winkel et al., 1976) looked at short-term biologic variation of serum proteins in healthy adults. Their main purpose was to estimate both intraindividual and interindividual physiological day-to-day variations in the constituents studied. Results of these investigations showed mean biological intraindividual variation to be much less than interindividual variation. These findings led them to suggest that, for specific proteins, baseline values obtained on an individual in good health would be useful in detecting changes in physiology before clinical manifestations became apparent. A similar study, performed over a period of 10 weeks with 700 apparently healthy adults, also found small intraindividual variations for IgG, IgA, IgM, and C3 (Butts et al., 1977). The relatively small intraindividual variations found in this study did not change when the population was divided according to age- and sex-groups.

C. Plasma Protein Patterns Typical of a Disorder

1. The Inflammatory Response

The general inflammatory response to active tissue turnover or necrosis is accompanied by characteristic plasma protein changes. These changes are coordinated with the time course of the inflammatory process, and may be used to differentiate between acute, subacute, and chronic pathological conditions. The intensity of the protein changes may or may not reflect the extent of tissue damage, and little is known concerning the mechanism that controls the acute phase response.

a. Postsurgical Acute Phase Response. Protein alterations resulting from surgical trauma have been investigated by several groups (Werner, 1969; Aronsen et al., 1972; Dickson and Alper, 1974; Fischer and Gill, 1975; Fischer et al., 1976). Surgery provides an excellent opportunity to study sequential protein changes with the time of trauma well established. In addition, the extent of tissue damage can be estimated and

TABLE II[a]

Postsurgical Acute Phase Response

Protein	6–8 hours	12 hours	1 day	2–3 days	1 week
Prealbumin			↓	↓↓	↓
Albumin			↓	↓	↓
α-Lipoprotein				↓	↓
α₁-Acid glycoprotein		↑	↑↑	↑↑↑	↑↑
α₁-Antitrypsin			↑	↑↑	↑
α₁-Antichymotrypsin	↑	↑	↑↑	↑↑↑	↑↑
α₂-Macroglobulin					
Ceruloplasmin					↑
Haptoglobin			↑	↑↑	↑
Hemopexin					↑
Gc-globulin					↑
Transferrin			↓	↓↓	↓
C3					↑
Fibrinogen			↑	↑↑	↑
IgG					
IgA					
IgM					
C-reactive protein	↑	↑	↑↑	↑↑↑	↑

[a] From Killingsworth, L. M. (1979). Plasma protein patterns in health and disease. *Crit. Rev. Clin. Lab. Sci.* **11**, 1–30. Reproduced by permission of the copyright owner.

complications can be kept to a minimum in a controlled setting. After uncomplicated surgery, C-reactive protein and α₁-antichymotrypsin rise within 6–8 h followed shortly by α₁-acid glycoprotein. These components reach maximum levels within 48–72 h. Strong reactions by α₁-antitrypsin, haptoglobin, and fibrinogen are observed at 24 h. Within 1 week moderate increases are seen with hemopexin, C3, ceruloplasmin, and Gc-globulin. Decreases in prealbumin, albumin, transferrin, and α-lipoprotein are seen in the first few postoperative days. Immunoglobulins show no response in the absence of infection or increased antigenic stimulation. α₂-Macroglobulin shows no response and, therefore, may serve as a control protein to monitor changes in hydrational status and blood volume. One exception to this finding is in bone surgery where α₂-macroglobulin levels have been shown to decrease early in the postoperative period (Dickson and Alper, 1974). Table II summarizes the acute phase response in uncomplicated surgery.

b. Acute Phase Response in Myocardial Infarction. The time of onset of myocardial infarction can be documented in many cases. Thus this disease process also lends itself to time-course studies of the acute phase proteins (Owen, 1967; Johansson *et al.*, 1972; Scherer and Ruhenstroth-Bauer, 1976; Smith *et al.*, 1977). Attempts have been made to correlate the extent of tissue injury in myocardial infarction with changes in the concentration of acute phase reactants. The general pattern consists of three phases. Rapid increases with a maximum at about 5 days for C-reactive protein, α_1-acid glycoprotein, α_1-antitrypsin, α_1-antichymotrypsin, haptoglobin, and fibrinogen with partial return to normal levels within 3 weeks. Prealbumin, albumin, transferrin, α-lipoprotein, and IgG show rapid decreases to a minimum at day 5 with return to normal in 3 weeks. Ceruloplasmin and C3 show moderate increases, which maximize during the second week. Only slight changes are observed for hemopexin, C4, α_2-macroglobulin, and IgM.

Johansson *et al.* (1972) could find no correlation between maximal enzyme levels and the intensity of the acute phase response. Smith and colleagues (1977), however, reported a quantitative relationship between enzymatic infarct size and the response of C-reactive protein, α_1-acid glycoprotein, haptoglobin, and fibrinogen. They theorized that humoral factors originating at the site of infarction were responsible for evoking increased protein synthesis by the liver.

c. Other Diseases. Ganrot (1974) studied acute phase proteins in three acute infectious diseases: peritonsillitis, serous meningoencephalitis, and influenza A. He found that α_1-acid glycoprotein, α_1-antichymotrypsin, α_1-antitrypsin, and haptoglobin exhibited marked increases in each disease when compared with levels after recovery. In influenza A, the mean level of C3 was not increased, and increases in C4 and ceruloplasmin were only moderate. Peritonsillitis led to increases in C-reactive protein, which were much higher than those observed in the other two diseases.

Fischer and Gill (1975) studied a panel of acute phase proteins (C-reactive protein, α_1-acid glycoprotein, α_1-antitrypsin, and haptoglobin) in infectious diseases. They found that the highest levels of all four proteins are observed with bacterial infections whereas viral infections resulted in relatively low levels of C-reactive protein and α_1-acid glycoprotein with moderate elevations in α_1-antitrypsin and haptoglobin.

Weeke and Jarnum (1971) investigated patients with Crohn's disease and ulcerative colitis, and found no significant differences between the protein patterns in the two diseases. Their studies showed increased serum concentrations of α_1-acid glycoprotein, α_1-antitrypsin, α_1-antichymotrypsin, haptoglobin, and hemopexin with decreased levels of prealbumin, albumin, ceruloplasmin, α_2-macroglobulin, and transferrin.

They concluded that concentrations of the positive acute phase reactants and immunoglobulins reflected the amount of disease activity.

Fischer and Gill (1975) showed that tumors which cause tissue necrosis can bring about a typical acute phase response. It can be characterized by low levels of C-reactive protein with marked elevations in α_1-acid glycoprotein and moderate increases in α_1-antitrypsin and haptoglobin. They pointed out, however, that the pattern was not diagnostic, and that a knowledge of the clinical circumstances would be essential for interpretation.

2. Rheumatic Diseases

The rheumatic diseases are characterized by both acute and chronic inflammatory episodes. This inflammation usually involves the connective tissues, but can be accompanied by systemic manifestations. Patients with rheumatic diseases frequently demonstrate plasma protein changes resulting from the acute inflammatory response and chronic stimulation of the immune system.

a. Rhematoid Arthritis. This is a chronic disease in which inflammation of the diarthroidal joints is often combined with a variety of extra-articular symptoms. Several investigators have studied either immunoglobulin levels or complete protein profiles in rheumatoid arthritis (Claman and Merrill, 1966; Barden *et al.*, 1967; Veys and Claessens, 1968; Pruzanski *et al.*, 1973; Killingsworth *et al.*, 1975b; Weiss, 1975; Watkins *et al.*, 1976). Immunoglobulin increases are most often of the IgA class with elevations in IgG and IgM occurring less often. No significant correlation has been shown between duration or stage of the disease and serum immunoglobulin levels. Though no distinct protein pattern is associated with rheumatoid arthritis, inflammatory protein patterns are commonly seen with α_1-acid glycoprotein, haptoglobin, and C3 as the most consistently abnormal components.

b. Juvenile Rheumatoid Arthritis. Goel and co-workers (1974) studied serum immunoglobulins and C3 in patients with juvenile rheumatoid arthritis. Though no correlation was found between levels of these proteins and severity or clinical course of the disease, a positive correlation did exist between immunoglobulin values and the severity of radiological changes. Anastassea-Vlachou *et al.* (1973) found significant elevations in haptoglobin and decreases in α_2-macroglobulin in children with juvenile arthritis when compared with age-matched healthy controls.

c. Systemic Lupus Erythematosus. Even though no specific pattern exists for this autoimmune disease, it can result in a wide variety of protein abnormalities (Alper, 1974; Killingsworth *et al.*, 1975b). The active disease process can produce a marked acute phase response, often with a normal or decreased haptoglobin due to *in vivo* hemolysis. Complement components C3 and C4 can be decreased in concentration due to activation of the complement system by circulating immune complexes. Immunoglobulins are commonly involved, with a cathodal increase in IgG being a characteristic, but not a diagnostic, finding. This protein pattern is summarized in Table III.

3. Liver Diseases

The liver is the primary organ for synthesis of most plasma proteins, the immunoglobulins being a notable exception. The Kupffer cells of the liver are, however, involved in the immune response in that they process antigens absorbed from the gut. As a consequence, disorders involving the liver can result in abnormalities of virtually all the plasma proteins.

a. Hepatitis. Kindmark and Laurell (1972) and Kindmark (1976) carried out extensive studies on patients with hepatitis A and B. They

TABLE III[a,b]

Systemic Lupus Erythematosus

Prealbumin	↓
Albumin	↓
α_1-Acid glycoprotein	↑
α_1-Antitrypsin	↑
α_2-Macroglobulin	N
Haptoglobin	N or ↓
Transferrin	↓
Complement C3	↓ or N
Complement C4	↓ or N
Fibrinogen	↑
IgG	↑ ↑ (cathodal)
IgA	N
IgM	N

[a] From Killingsworth, L. M. (1979). Plasma protein patterns in health and disease. *Crit. Rev. Clin. Lab. Sci.* **11,** 1–30. Reproduced by permission of the copyright owner.

[b] This is the pattern seen with active disease: including acute and chronic inflammation with stimulation of the immune system, *in vivo* hemolysis, and complement consumption.

showed that the characteristic acute phase response was not present with either disease, but that specific patterns for some acute phase reactants did occur. In hepatitis B they found that α_1-antitrypsin was increased from the beginning with elevations persisting during the first month of illness. Values for α_1-acid glycoprotein clustered around the normal mean and haptoglobin levels were below the normal mean during the first month.

Their results for hepatitis A revealed increased levels of α_1-acid glycoprotein for the first 10 days of the disease and elevations of haptoglobin above the normal mean for the first 2 weeks. They concluded that measurements of α_1-antitrypsin, α_1-acid glycoprotein, and haptoglobin can be useful in the differential diagnosis of hepatitis during the first 2 weeks of illness.

Their findings for immunoglobulins in hepatitis B showed elevations of IgM with a maximum during the first week and a gradual return to normal. Levels of IgA and IgG were generally found to be normal in hepatitis B. Increases of IgM were much greater in hepatitis A than in hepatitis B, and showed large individual variations. Values for IgA and IgG were slightly higher in patients with hepatitis A for the first 2 weeks and 1 week, respectively. Due to large individual variations, the authors felt that immunoglobulin levels were of little utility in the differential diagnosis of hepatitis A and B. No significant difference between the two diseases was found for albumin, α-lipoprotein, α_1-antichymotrypsin, ceruloplasmin, hemopexin, transferrin, C3, C4, fibrinogen, plasminogen, prothrombin, and C-reactive protein. Prealbumin, however, was seen to be a reliable indicator of the clinical course for both hepatitis A and B. Other investigators have confirmed the value of prealbumin as a sensitive indicator of liver function by showing a progressive decrease of this protein during the passage from chronic persistent hepatitis, to chronic aggressive hepatitis, to postnecrotic cirrhosis in viral liver disease (Agostoni *et al.*, 1974, 1976).

b. Cirrhosis. In the cirrhotic process, both the ability of the liver to synthesize proteins and the effectiveness of Kuppfer cells to process antigens can be compromised. Studies of patients with alcoholic and cryptogenic cirrhosis reflect both these pathophysiological circumstances (Lo-Grippo *et al.*, 1971; Hällén *et al.*, 1972; Bouige *et al.*, 1973; Hiramatsu *et al.*, 1976). The pattern most commonly observed included diffuse increases in IgG with proportionally greater increases in IgA and, less frequently, increases in IgM. Of the positive acute phase reactants, α_1-antitrypsin was the most sensitive indicator for hepatocellular disease whereas C-reactive protein, ceruloplasmin, and fibrinogen were usually normal or slightly increased. Levels of α_1-acid glycoprotein were normal

TABLE IV[a]

Cirrhosis

Prealbumin	↓
Albumin	↓
α-Lipoprotein	↓
α_1-Acid glycoprotein	N or ↓
α_1-Antitrypsin	↑ ↑
α_2-Macroglobulin	↑
Ceruloplasmin	N or ↑
Haptoglobin	N or ↓
Transferrin	↓
C3	N or ↓
Fibrinogen	N or ↑
IgG	↑
IgA	↑ ↑
IgM	N or ↑
C-reactive protein	N or ↑

[a] From Killingsworth, L. M. (1979). Plasma protein patterns in health and disease. *Crit. Rev. Clin. Lab. Sci.* **11**, 1–30. Reproduced by permission of the copyright owner.

or decreased. Haptoglobin was usually normal but could be decreased as a result of hemolysis or reduced hepatic blood flow. Complement component C3 was usually normal but advanced cirrhosis could lead to decreased synthesis and subnormal levels. The negative acute phase reactants, prealbumin, albumin, α-lipoprotein, and transferrin showed characteristic decreases with prealbumin indicated as the most sensitive monitor of hepatic function in cirrhosis. Concentrations of α_2-macroglobulin were significantly elevated in cirrhosis. The general pattern for alcoholic cirrhosis is summarized in Table IV.

MacSween and co-workers (1972) investigated serum proteins in patients with primary biliary cirrhosis and compared results with age- and sex-matched controls. They demonstrated decreases in albumin levels, increases in α_2-macroglobulin, IgG, IgA, and IgM, with no significant changes in transferrin and C3. No significant correlations were found between the proteins assayed and either antimitochondrial antibody titer or duration of symptoms.

c. Obstructive Jaundice. LoGrippo and co-workers (1971) studied patients with extrahepatic biliary obstruction. They found normal levels of IgG with normal levels of IgM, except in rare instances where there was inflammation associated with obstruction. Slight, but frequent, elevations in IgA were observed. Albumin decreases were noted along with increases in ceruloplasmin, transferrin, and C-reactive protein. Complement C3 levels were found to be normal, decreased, and increased. Alper (1974) has commented that "pure" biliary obstruction is associated with increases in C3 and β-lipoprotein. Bouige *et al.* (1973) observed elevations of α_1-acid glycoprotein, α_1-antitrypsin, and haptoglobin in this disorder. These diverse findings are a result, in part, of different proteins studied by the various groups. The amount of inflammation associated with the obstructive process could also be an important consideration.

4. Protein-Losing Disorders

a. Selective Protein Loss. Nephrosis and some protein-losing gastroenteropathies can result in loss of proteins in an inverse relationship to their molecular weight or, more accurately, their hydrodynamic volume (Joachim *et al.*, 1964; MacLean and Robson, 1967; Hardwicke *et al.*, 1970; Weeke *et al.* 1971a,b; Henry, 1974). This leads to elevations in the concentrations of large proteins—absolute elevations, since the rate of hepatic protein synthesis is increased—with decreases in smaller components. The serum pattern, shown in Table V, shows increased levels of

TABLE V[a,b]

Selective Protein Loss

Prealbumin	↓
Albumin	↓
α_1-Acid glycoprotein	↓
α_1-Antitrypsin	↓
α_2-Macroglobulin	↑ ↑
Haptoglobin	↑ or ↓
Transferrin	↓
β-Lipoprotein	↑ ↑
IgG	↓
IgA	N or ↓
IgM	↑

[a] From Killingsworth, L. M. (1979). Plasma protein patterns in health and disease. *Crit. Rev. Clin. Lab. Sci.* **11**, 1–30. Reproduced by permission of the copyright owner.

[b] Haptoglobin loss depends on genetic type; absolute elevations are seen with large proteins.

α_2-macroglobulin, β-lipoprotein, and polymeric forms of haptoglobin (Hp 2-1 and Hp2-2) with decreases in such proteins as prealbumin, albumin, α_1-acid glycoprotein, α_1-antitrypsin, and transferrin. Immunoglobulin M is usually elevated in relation to the small proteins, and IgG is usually decreased. Loss of lymphatic fluid in protein-losing enteropathies can result in decreased levels of IgG, IgA, and IgM (Ritzmann, 1975).

b. Nonselective Protein Loss. A diminished capacity of the glomerulus to act as a molecular sieve, nonselective gastrointestinal protein-loss, or whole blood loss, can lead to diffuse hypoproteinemia in the plasma (Joachim *et al.*, 1964; MacLean and Robson, 1967; Hardwicke *et al.*, 1970). It should be noted this protein pattern can also result from congestive heart failure, liver failure, hemodilution, and malnutrition.

5. Pregnancy and Hyperestrogenism

Ganrot (1972) studied protein profiles in normal pregnancy and compared them with values found in healthy, nonpregnant women. He found that haptoglobin and C3 showed mean concentrations within $\pm 10\%$ of the corresponding values for nonpregnant women. Prealbumin, albumin, α_1-acid glycoprotein, and IgG were moderately decreased in pregnant women. The α_1-acid glycoprotein decrease is confirmed by other studies (Adams and Wacher, 1968). Large relative increases were found for α_1-antitrypsin, ceruloplasmin, transferrin, and fibrinogen. Values for α-lipoprotein were increased to a moderate degree whereas α_2-macroglobulin and hemopexin were slightly elevated in the group of pregnant women. This pattern takes on added significance when considering that estrogen medication, including contraceptive pills, can produce hyperestrogenism. The pregnancy or "pseudopregnancy" pattern can be thus superimposed over pathological changes in young women taking contraceptive pills or others on estrogen medication. Milford-Ward and colleagues (1976) assayed α_1-fetoprotein in maternal serum in an effort to avoid amniocentesis when screening for fetal neural tract abnormalities. They concluded that raised maternal serum α_1-fetoprotein levels could be used as a parameter to identify a pregnancy "at risk" and as an indicator for follow-up studies such as amniocentesis.

Burnett and colleagues (1976) assessed plasma protein profiles in normal pregnancy as compared with pre-eclampsia. They found that the only significant protein change was a decrease in transferrin with severe pre-eclampsia.

Forkman *et al.* (1972) determined the plasma concentrations of 17 proteins in a series of women with recurrent cholestasis of pregnancy and in a control series of normal pregnant women. The protein pattern found in recurrent cholestasis showed primarily mild changes characteristic of hepatocellular damage and biliary obstruction.

6. Plasma Cell Dyscrasias

Plasma cell dyscrasias—also known as monoclonal gammopathies, immunocytomas, and paraimmunoglobulinopathies—are characterized by an excessive proliferation of a single clone of plasma cells leading to the production of large quantities of one homogenous immunoglobulin (Heremans and Masson, 1973; Quittner, 1974; Ritzmann, 1975). Ritzmann (1975) has defined plasma cell dyscrasias as being associated with (a) excessive and often neoplastic proliferation of B-lymphocyte clones, usually without apparent antigenic stimulus; (b) synthesis of homogenous immunoglobulins or immunoglobulin subunits; and (c) frequently, decreased levels of the normal immunoglobulins. These disorders can present a dramatic pattern-a sharply demarcated, intense band on electrophoresis and elevation of one immunoglobulin with decreased levels of the others—but often the protein manifestations are not so clearcut. It should also be noted that even though the majority of patients with immunochemical evidence of plasma cell dyscrasia are symptomatic; one-third of patients with monoclonal proteins are asymptomatic (Ritzmann, 1975). These circumstances make it of paramount importance that the laboratory investigate possible plasma cell dyscrasias with a variety of analytical techniques and carry out close consultation with the attending physician. Electrophoretic and immunoelectrophoretic (or immunofixation) studies of urine and serum samples should be coupled with quantitative immunochemical analysis. These quantitative measurements of the monoclonal protein over a period of time could aid in the differential diagnosis of benign or malignant plasma cell dyscrasias and could provide useful information concerning the rate of growth of the tumor clone.

7. Genetic Deficiencies

a. α_1-Antitrypsin. This protein exhibits complex polymorphism, which is described by the Pi (protease inhibitor) system. Individuals with a severe deficiency of α_1-antitrypsin show an increased susceptibility to hepatic disease, from portal fibrosis to cirrhosis, and lung disorders, from bronchopulmonary symptoms to panlobular emphysema (Gitlin and Gitlin, 1975b; Daniels, 1975b; Janus and Carrell, 1976). It should be noted that α_1-antitrypsin is a positive acute phase reactant. The synthetic stimulus of inflammation should be considered and evaluated when screening for α_1-antitrypsin deficiency.

b. Complement Components. Deficiencies of most components of the complement sequence have been described (Gitlin and Gitlin, 1975b; Tucker and Nakamura, 1975; Müller-Eberhard, 1975; Whicher, 1978). These conditions are not common and usually result in the total absence of a single component. Patients with complement deficiencies may present with increased susceptibility to infection or a wide range of other symptoms.

c. Immunoglobulins. Immunodeficiency diseases are those conditions in which the immune system fails to function properly *in vivo,* and are clinically characterized by recurrent infections (Ritzmann, 1975). Deficiencies in the humoral antibody response can lead to decreased levels of one or more of the immunoglobulins. With agammaglobulinemia or hypogammaglobulinemia, the serum levels of all major immunoglobulins are decreased. This condition is seen in the transient hypogammaglobulinemia of infancy and in several conditions classified under the heading of variable immunodeficiency. Deficiencies of one or two major classes of immunoglobulins give rise to a constellation of disorders known as dysgammaglobulinemias. The majority of patients with immunoglobulin deficiencies cannot be satisfactorily classified, and are designated as variable immunodeficiencies.

d. Other Proteins. Genetic deficiencies of other proteins are not common, but include albumin, haptoglobin, transferrin, cholinesterase, fibrinogen, coagulation factors, α_1-antichymotrypsin, α-lipoprotein, and β-lipoprotein (Daniels, 1975a; Gitlin and Gitlin, 1975b; Peters, 1975; Putnam, 1975a,b). Decreased levels of ceruloplasmin are observed in Wilson's disease, but this is probably not due to a genetic inability to synthesize the protein (Poulik and Weiss, 1975).

D. Reporting Protein Profile Data

One approach to protein profile reporting is depicted in Fig. 2. The graphical section of the report contains columns for charting results. The scale of the graph has been adjusted to produce reference intervals of equal size for all proteins. When colored lines representing patient data are drawn on the graph, results above and below the reference intervals

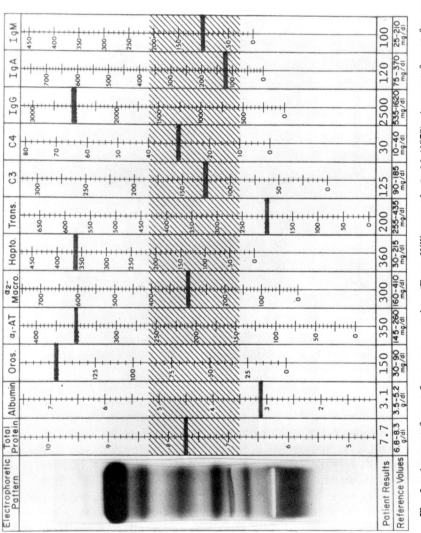

Fig. 2. A report format for serum proteins. (From Killingsworth, L. M. (1978). A report format for serum proteins, *Clin. Chem.* **24,** 728. Reproduced by permission of the copyright owner.)

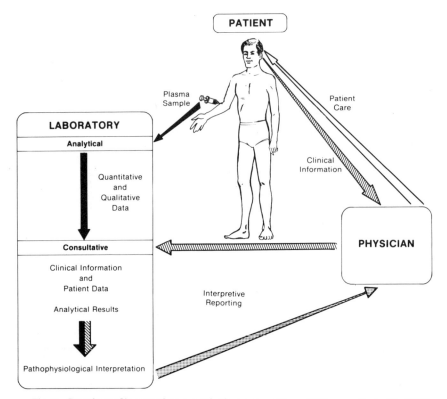

Fig. 3. Protein profile reporting: a synthetic process. (From Killingsworth, L. M. (1979). Plasma protein patterns in health and disease. *Crit. Rev. Clin. Lab. Sci.* **11,** 1–30. Reproduced by permission of the copyright owner.)

are easily detected. Plotting data in this manner results in characteristic and easily recognizable patterns for various pathophysiological conditions. Attachment of a photograph of the agarose gel electrophoretic pattern gives a broad overview of the patient's protein status and reinforces the quantitative data. Spaces are provided at the bottom of the report sheet for numerical results.

Further condensation of the data can result from interpretive comments inserted in a section on clinical considerations. In this area the laboratory director can provide a valuable service by commenting on significant findings. This is a synthetic and consultative exercise, as shown in Fig. 3, where pertinent information from the history and physical examination are considered along with specific protein results and other laboratory data to produce an overall pathophysiological commentary.

II. CEREBROSPINAL FLUID PROTEINS

A. Overview of CSF Proteins

Cerebrospinal fluid is formed through ultrafiltration of plasma in the highly vascularized choroid plexus of the lareral, third, and fourth ventricles (Schultze and Heremans, 1966b). The molecular sieve effect in the choroid plexuses produces a clear fluid with relatively low protein content. Ventricular CSF has a lower protein content than fluid drawn from the lumbar region. In addition, newborns and elderly patients exhibit higher CSF protein levels than individuals in other age-groups. Lumbar CSF from normal adults is generally considered to contain from 15–65 mg of protein per deciliter.

The protein composition of cerebrospinal fluid is similar to serum except that the relative content of low molecular weight proteins is greater in CSF (Laurell, 1972a). Electrophoresis of 100-fold concentrated CSF from normal individuals results in a pattern with a prominent prealbumin fraction which migrates slightly on the anodal side of its plasma counterpart. Also of note in the CSF electrophoretic pattern are relative decreases in large proteins such as α_2-macroglobulin and polymeric haptoglobin phenotypes. Transferrin is detected in the β_1-region and the β_2-region is dominated by a slowly migrating "CSF-specific" transferrin. Some slight banding is present in the γ-region and the cathodal end of this zone often contains a low molecular weight, nonimmunoglobulin in "γ-trace" protein.

Studies on specific cerebrospinal fluid proteins in disease have concentrated on assessment of blood–CSF interface permeability changes and quantitation of abnormal protein production within the CNS. Permeability increases are observed in a wide variety of disorders, whereas increased synthesis of CSF immunoglobulin is associated with demyelinating processes and other inflammatory CNS diseases. Some neurological diseases exhibit CSF patterns which are characterized by permeability changes combined with increased immunoglobulin production.

B. Use of CSF Protein Data in the Diagnosis of Neurological Disease

1. Demyelinating Diseases

Kabat and co-workers (1948) demonstrated in 1948 that the cerebrospinal fluid of some patients with multiple sclerosis contained elevated levels of γ-globulin. Since that time, numerous groups have searched for more sensitive and specific laboratory measurements to aid in the diagnosis of demyelinating diseases (Schneck and Claman, 1969; Riddoch and Thompson, 1970; Link and Muller, 1971; Tourtellotte *et al.*, 1971; Berner *et al.*, 1972; Savory and Heintges, 1973; Skrabanek *et al.*, 1973; Ganrot and Laurell, 1974; Perry *et al.*, 1974; Schliep and Felgenhauer, 1974; Ansari *et al.*, 1975; Lamoureux *et al.*, 1975; Delpech and Boquet, 1976; Britain *et al.*, 1977).

Quantitative immunochemical studies have shown that the increased CSF γ-globulin content in demyelinating diseases is due to increased synthesis of IgG within the CNS. The specific antigenic stimulant for the IgG production is unclear, but mechanisms involving both viral infection and autoimmunity have been proposed (Adams and Dickinson, 1974). It should be noted that increased levels of CSF IgG are not specific for demyelinating diseases, since they are also observed in other inflammatory CNS disorders such as neurosyphilis and CNS lupus (Schneck and Claman, 1969; Riddoch and Thompson, 1970; Link and Muller, 1971; Savory and Heintges, 1973; Skrabanek *et al.*, 1973; Britain *et al.*, 1977). Elevations of IgA and IgM are infrequently observed in demyelinating diseases, but are of negligible diagnostic value (Schneck and Claman, 1969; Riddoch and Thompson, 1970; Link and Muller, 1971; Savory and Heintges, 1973).

Evaluation of CSF IgG levels must take into consideration the condition of the blood–CSF interface, since increases resulting from leakage of serum proteins across the interface must be differentiated from increased CNS production. One method of taking the permeability factor into account is to calcualte CSF IgG as a percentage of CSF total protein (Schneck and Claman, 1969; Riddoch and Thompson, 1970; Link and Muller, 1971; Berner *et al.*, 1972; Savory and Heintges, 1973; Skrabanek *et al.*, 1973; Ansari *et al.*, 1975; Lamoureux *et al.*, 1975). Even though the upper limits of normal for this fraction, as reported by several groups from data on healthy adult controls, do not agree exactly, deviation from a mean value of 11.3% is slight in most cases. Levels of 10% are generally considered suspicious, with levels greater than 13% suggestive of increased IgG production.

Tourtellotte *et al.* (1971) demonstrated that the ratio of CSF IgG/CSF albumin was as discriminative for multiple sclerosis as the CSF IgG/CSF total protein ratio. They found the range in normal adults to be 17.1% ± 8.2. Perry and colleagues (1974) studied methods for determining CSF IgG/CSF albumin ratios, and found electroimmunoassay to be superior to radial immunodiffusion in precision. This is an important factor when calculating the ratio of two parameters. Schliep and Felgenhauer (1974) chose CSF α_2-macroglobulin to indicate the condition of the blood–CSF interface, and showed that the ratio CSF IgG/CSF α_2-macroglobulin could be used to discriminate between patients with multiple sclerosis and those with other neurological diseases such as spinal tumors and meningitis.

Ganrot and Laurell (1974) showed that the predictive value of CSF protein measurements could be improved if serum proteins were also taken into consideration. They chose albumin as a reference protein to provide information about permeability of the blood–CSF interface and CSF protein turnover. The ratio CSF IgG/serum IgG normalized data on this protein for serum levels. When these two ratios were displayed graphically, a clear separation could be seen between patients with increased production of IgG and normal permeability (e.g., multiple sclerosis), those with only increased blood–CSF interface permeability and those with combined disorders. Delpech and Boquet (1976) published a "K value" to represent the ratio of the two ratios previously discussed.

$$K = \frac{\text{CSF IgG/CSF albumin}}{\text{Serum IgG/serum albumin}}$$

Their results for normal subjects showed a mean value of $0.52^{\pm} 0.32$ (2 S.D.). This mathematical reduction of the graphical presentation of Ganrot and Laurell (1974) allowed for a more quantitative evaluation of patient data. Britain *et al.* (1977) employed the dual ratio approach and reported data similar to that of Delpech and Boquet for healthy individuals. They calculated a K value of 0.50 (range 0.34–0.66) and included parameters for a graphical reference area. Figure 4 illustrates the reference area, enclosed in the dashed lines, generated from data on 47 healthy controls. The control data had the following characteristics: slope of the reference line 0.588, y intercept -4.0×10^{-4}, and standard error of estimate 7.0×10^{-4}. Nonparametric statistical evaluation of the CSF data produced normal ranges of 0.5–9.5 mg/dl for IgG and 5.0–50.0 mg/dl for albumin. Clinical studies on patients with multiple sclerosis and other neurological diseases are presented in Fig. 5. Eight of the nine multiple sclerosis patients had ratio values in the area of the graph representing increased CNS production of IgG with normal permeability. Patients with nondemyelinating neurological diseases generally fell within the multivariant reference area or showed "pure" permeability increases.

Electrophoretic studies of CSF from patients with demyelinating diseases have shown a characteristic pattern of oligoclonal banding in the γ region in a high percentage of cases (Laterre *et al.*, 1970; Link, 1973; Johnson *et al.*, 1977). These multiple bands of restricted electrophoretic heterogeneity can be detected on agarose gel elctrophoresis of concen-

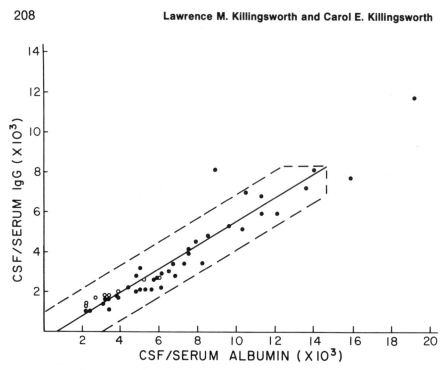

Fig. 4. Reference area for CSF/serum specific protein ratios. Open circles, children; closed circles, adults. (From Britain *et al.* (1977). CSF/serum protein ratios in the diagnosis of neurological disease. *In* "Advances in Automated Analysis" (E. C. Barton *et al.,* eds.), pp. 274–277. Mediad, New York. Reproduced by permission of the copyright owner.)

trated CSF, but a comparison should be made with the paitents' serum pattern to rule out the possibility of oligoclonal or monoclonal serum bands. As with quantitative IgG studies, oligoclonal bands have been observed in some nondemyelinating inflammatory CNS diseases. Cohen and co-workers (1976), in an attempt to provide a specific laboratory test for demyelination, have developed a radioimmunoassay procedure to determine myelin basic protein in CSF. Their studies showed that patients with active demyelinating diseases had high levels of myelin basic protein (17–100 ng/ml) whereas patients with slowly progressive multiple sclerosis had intermediate values (6–16 ng/ml) and those in remission had low values (less than 4 ng/ml). The determination of myelin basic protein thus shows promise both as an index for diagnosis of demyelinating diseases and as a parameter for following the clinical course of these disorders.

2. Disorders Associated with Increased Blood–CSF Interface Permeability

Many CNS disorders cause increases in the permeability of the blood–CSF interface, leading to elevated CSF protein levels. Among

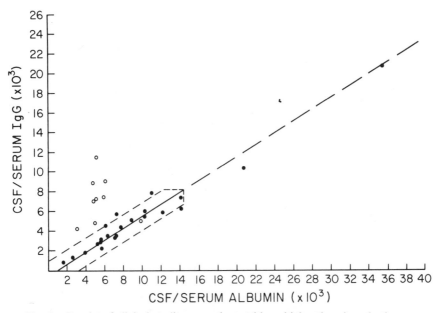

Fig. 5. Results of clinical studies on patients with multiple sclerosis and other neurological diseases. Open circles, multiple sclerosis; closed circles, other neurological diseases. (From Britain *et al.* (1977). CSF/serum specific protein ratios in the diagnosis of neurological disease. *In* "Advances in Automated Analysis" (E. C. Barton *et al.*, eds.), pp. 274–277. Mediad, New York. Reproduced by permission of the copyright owner.)

these are included all types of meningitis, neoplastic infiltrations of the meninges, spinal and cerebral tumors, polyneuropathies, disk herniations, and cerebral infarctions (Schneck and Claman, 1969; Laterre *et al.*, 1970; Riddoch and Thompson, 1970; Link and Muller, 1971; O'Toole *et al.*, 1971; Savory and Heintges, 1973; Skrabanek *et al.*, 1973; Smith *et al.*, 1973; Britain *et al.*, 1977). In conditions that are characterized by infection or antigenic stimulation, elevations of one or more immunoglobulins can be superimposed over the general hyperproteinemia. Elevations of IgG are most common, followed by IgA, and, more rarely, IgM.

Several groups have assessed blood–CSF interface permeability through measurement of CSF proteins or CSF/serum protein ratios. Britain *et al.* (1977) showed that "pure" permeability increases led to elevated values of both the ratios CSF IgG/serum IgG and CSF albumin/serum albumin in proportions which caused patient points to fall on or very close to their calculated permeability line. Examples of this are the two points near the line represented by longer dashes in Fig. 5. They also reported that patients with "combined disorders," such as chronic bacterial meningitis, generally gave ratio values which illustrated both increased permeability and increased CNS IgG production.

Schliep and Felgenhauer (1974) proposed the quantitation of a high molecular weight protein in CSF, α_2-macroglobulin, as a method for evaluation of the condition of the blood–CSF interface. They showed that the relative proportions of passively transferred proteins and those synthesized within the CNS could be evaluated in this manner. Their studies indicated that the α_2-macroglobulin level in CSF was a more sensitive indicator for mild interface disturbances than the total protein content. They also investigated changes in the protein content of CSF during the course of bacterial meningitis. Initial complete interface breakdown, illustrated by increased levels of α_2-macroglobulin and normal relative amounts of IgG, was followed by a healing stage as interface permeability returned toward normal (decreasing α_2-macroglobulin) and the immune response was activated (increasing IgG).

Felgenhauer and co-workers (1976) performed extensive studies on protein size and CSF composition. They concluded that many proteins showed fundamental differences between their hydrodynamic volume and molecular weight, and that the volume factor was critical in determining CSF protein composition. They plotted serum/CSF protein concentration ratios against hydrodynamic volume for albumin, ceruloplasmin, and α_2-macroglobulin as a means of assessing blood–CSF interface permeability. Ratios for these three proteins constitute a straight-line relationship with molecular size, thus the determination of cereuloplasmin could be omitted in routine applications.

III. URINE PROTEINS OF PLASMA ORIGIN

A. Overview of Urine Proteins

Filtration of plasma across the glomerular capillary membrane, the initial event in the formation of urine, produces fluid containing a greatly reduced content of proteins with molecular weights in excess of 40,000. Plasma proteins of small size are normally filtered almost freely through the glomeruli, and are subsequently reabsorbed by the renal tubules. Normal urinary protein excretion, therefore, is less than 150 mg/day (Schultze and Heremans, 1966a; Hardwicke, 1970; Lambert et al., 1970; Laurell, 1972a; Hardwicke, 1974; Heinemann, 1974; Killingsworth et al., 1975a). Two-thirds of this is made up of filtered plasma proteins, the remainder being derived from the urinary tract itself (Boyce et al., 1961).

Immunochemical methods have allowed detection of numerous plasma proteins in normal urine and have shown albumin and IgG to be quantitatively dominant (Berggard, 1961; Berggard and Risinger, 1961; Rowe and

Soothill, 1961; Poortmans and Jeanloz, 1968; Berggard, 1970; Weeke, 1974; Hemmingsen and Skaarup, 1975; Ellis and Buffone, 1977). The extensive investigations of Hemmingsen and Skaarup (1975) showed a wide and uneven distribution of urine protein excretion, characterized by many points clustered at low levels with much "tailing" of data toward higher values. They also found large physiological day-to-day variations for excretion of several proteins in a healthy subject. This finding is in striking contrast to the small physiological variations reported for proteins in plasma (Statland et al., 1976; Winkel et al., 1976; Butts et al., 1977).

Estimation of protein in urine has long been used in the evaluation of kidney diseases. The importance of making quantitative urinary albumin measurements was recognized as early as 1914 when Folin and Denis (1914) reported a procedure utilizing sulphosalicylic acid. Since that time, the advent of electrophoretic and immunochemical procedures has helped bring about a clearer understanding of the mechanisms of proteinuria in renal and systemic disorders.

Proteinuria in renal disease can be classified as resulting from either glomerular or tubular dysfunction. Glomerular proteinuria results from increased transcapillary passage of proteins through the glomerulus and is characterized by the loss of plasma proteins the size of albumin or larger (Blainey et al., 1960; Schultze and Heremans, 1966a; Maiorca et al., 1967; Trip et al., 1968; Peterson et al., 1969; Barratt et al., 1970; Hardwicke, 1970; Hardwicke et al., 1970; Revillard et al., 1970; Hardwicke, 1974; Heinemann et al., 1974; Hofer et al., 1974; Stuhlinger et al., 1974). Tubular proteinuria is caused by a decreased capacity of the tubules to reabsorb proteins. With normal glomerular function, the glomerular filtrate contains high concentrations of low molecular weight proteins to be reabsorbed by the tubules. Thus, impaired tubular function causes increased excretion of these small proteins (Friberg, 1950; Butler and Flynn, 1958; Butler et al., 1962; Schultze and Heremans, 1966a; Peterson et al., 1969; Hardwicke, 1970; Hardwicke et al., 1970; Laterre and Manual, 1970; Revillard et al., 1970b; Dillard et al., 1971; Hardwicke, 1974; Heinemann, 1974; Ravnskov and Johansson, 1974; Ricanti and Hall, 1974; Wibell and Evrin, 1974).

Certain systemic conditions, some of which are considered benign, others pathological, can lead to increased urinary protein excretion. These conditions include exercise proteinuria, postural proteinuria, proteinuria of pregnancy, febrile proteinuria, and overflow proteinuria (Schultze and Heremans, 1966a; Poortmans and Jeanloz, 1968; Charvet et al., 1970; Hardwicke, 1970; Hardwicke et al., 1970; Poortmans, 1970; Robinson, 1970; Hardwicke, 1974; Heinemann et al., 1974; Jensen and Henriksen, 1974; Poortmans, 1974).

B. Use of Urine Protein Data in the Assessment of Renal Function

1. Glomerular Proteinuria

A variety of pathological processes can cause glomerular injury resulting in proteinuria (Heinemann *et al.*, 1974). Heavy urinary protein loss may be associated with immune complex diseases such as systemic lupus erythematosus, poststreptococcal glomerulonephritis, and membranous glomerulonephritis. The deposition of abnormal substances such as occurs in amyloidosis or diabetic glomerulosclerosis can lead to increased glomerular permeability. Proteinuria is also observed in chronic pyelonephritis, as a result of some cardiovascular diseases, and some congenital renal abnormalities. Severe protein loss can occur with some renal diseases of unknown etiology such as lipoid nephrosis and idiopathic nephrotic syndrome.

The renal glomeruli, which function as ultrafilters, are considered to be membranes interrupted by pores of fixed dimensions which allow for passage of certain molecular species and retention of others (Hardwicke *et al.*, 1970; Heinemann *et al.*, 1974). Urine from patients with selective glomerular proteinuria (nephrotic syndrome) contains large amounts of albumin, α_1-antitrypsin, and transferrin, which are normally retained by the glomerulus.

Quantitative assessment of glomerular function can be carried out through measurement of the renal clearance of proteins with different molecular sizes (Blainey *et al.*, 1960; Maiorca *et al.*, 1967; Trip *et al.*, 1968; Revillard *et al.*, 1970a; Hofer *et al.*, 1974; Stuhlinger *et al.*, 1974). When relative protein clearance values are plotted against molecular weight on a double log scale, a linear relationship can be found through least squares analysis, though considerable scatter of the points is often observed. The slope of this line has been used to characterize the selectivity of the glomerulus to protein excretion. Though these determinations have limited usefulness in the classification of disease entities, several studies have shown that patients with selective nephrotic syndrome (slope > 67°) generally have a better prognosis and response to steroid therapy than do patients with nonselective protein loss.

The validity of the selectivity index was placed in some doubt, however, when Hofer *et al.* (1974) reported little prognostic value for selectivity data in their studies of glomerulonephritis. More recently, Ellis and Buffone (1977) showed that the selectivity index does not delineate between pathologically distinct disease states, and that the amount of a given protein in urine is not directly proportional to its molecular weight alone. Other factors that could influence protein passage through the glomerulus could include molecular charge, hydrodynamic radius of the protein, viscous drag, and protein–protein binding, as well as charge of the glomerular membrane and glomerular filtration rate (Heinemann *et al.*, 1974; Ellis and Buffone, 1977). The influence of these additional factors, which are not considered in calculation of the selectivity index, limits the usefulness of this concept and emphasizes the need for a new approach in the evaluation of a glomerular proteinuria.

2. Tubular Proteinuria

As shown by Friberg (1950), increased amounts of low molecular weight proteins appear in the urine of workers chronically exposed to cadmium dust. Butler and Flynn (1958) reported that the type of proteinuria found in patients with renal tubular dysfunction is markedly different from the proteinuria associated with glomerular damage. These findings have been confirmed in other studies which have demonstrated that the urine proteins of patients with renal tubular diseases have low sedimentation coefficients and electrophoretic mobilities mainly in the α_2 and β regions (Butler *et al.*, 1962; Laterre and Manuel, 1970; Revillard *et al.*, 1970b; Dillard *et al.*, 1971). Revillard *et al.* (1970b) found a strong correlation between the presence of tubular type proteinuria as defined by its biochemical characteristics, and the presence of tubular or interstitial disorders as defined histiologically or by other biological evidence. They suggested that tubular dysfunction could be studied through measurement of a characteristic urinary protein.

A physiological mechanism for tubular proteinuria was proposed by Schultze and Heremans (1966a) and was based on the assumption that low molecular weight proteins are filtered by the normal glomerulus to a much greater extent than proteins the size of albumin. They are thus available for tubular reabsorption in greater amounts than the larger proteins. Any decrease in the capacity of the tubules to reabsorb proteins, therefore, would be reflected to a greater extent in the increased excretion of small proteins.

The urinary protein most often studied in tubular proteinuria is β_2-microglobulin. This small protein (molecular weight 1100), first described by Berggard and Bearn (1968), exhibits striking structural homogeneity with regions of the light and heavy chains of immunoglobulins. Urinary excretion of β_2-microglobulin is at a rate of about 100 $\mu g/24$ h, and serum levels for adults range from 0.8 to 2.4 $\mu g/ml$ (Evrin and Wibell, 1972). The biological function of β_2-microglobulin is unknown, but its small size makes it suitable for studies of tubular reabsorptive function.

Peterson *et al.* (1969) suggested that quantitative determinations of urinary β_2-microglobulin and urinary albumin could be useful in differentiating between glomerular and tubular proteinuria. They pointed out, however, that mixed glomerular–tubular types are observed in patients with chronic renal failure and chronic pyelonephritis. Wibell and Evrin (1974) postulated a saturation point for tubular reabsorption of β_2-microglobulin at a serum level of about 4.5 μg/ml. They stated that at serum levels below this value, measurement of urinary β_2-microglobulin is probably a good estimator of tubular reabsorption. Other investigators (Ravnskov and Johansson, 1974) have suggested that β_2-microglobulin might also be eliminated by an extraglomerular mechanism, possibly by direct uptake from peritubular vessels. Ricanati and Hall (1974) studied serum β_2-microglobulin levels in the anuric phase following renal transplantation. They concluded that a progressive drop in serum β_2-microglobulin concentration during this period suggested a viable graft even in the absence of excretory renal function.

C. Other Conditions Associated with Increased Urine Protein Excretion

Several physiological conditions have been shown to produce proteinuria in the absence of significant renal disease. Studies have shown that strenuous muscular exercise produces a rise in the urinary excretion of both high and low molecular weight proteins (Poortmans and Jeanloz, 1968; Poortmans, 1970; Poortmans, 1974). It has been suggested by Poortmans (1974) that exercise proteinuria is mainly due to increased glomerular permeability combined with saturation or inhibition of tubular reabsorption capacity by some unknown mechanism.

Postural or orthostatic proteinuria is defined as a syndrome whose diagnosis requires both the absence of proteinuria during recumbency, and its presence when the patient is in an upright position. Postural proteinuria has long been regarded as a benign condition unassociated with renal disease, though some recent reports have contradicted this view (Robinson, 1970). Total daily protein excretion is usually well below 1.5 gm in this condition with relatively large percentages of high molecular weight proteins. Tentative mechanisms for postural proteinuria propose increased nonselective glomerular permeability on standing, but the underlying cause has not been characterized.

The proteinuria seen in pregnant women is usually transitory and does not indicate actual renal disease (Charvet et al., 1970). Proteinurias of pregnancy can be classified as proteinuria associated with toxemia, proteinuria during delivery, proteinuria during renal infections, and proteinuria with no other clinical symptoms. In proteinuria with toxemia, a selective pattern is usually associated with a high rate of fetal mortality *in utero*. Proteinuria during delivery conforms with a glomerular pattern in most cases. Though most urinary infections in pregnancy do not cause proteinuria, those that do can show nonselective or mixed tubular patterns. Proteinuria without clinical symptoms usually produces a nonselective pattern.

Jensen and Hendriksen (1974) studied the urinary excretion of specific proteins in patients with various nonrenal infectious diseases. They found abnormal urine protein excretion in almost all patients and postulted that "febrile proteinuria" results from temporary immunological injury to the glomerular basement membrane caused by deposition of antigen–antibody complexes.

Increased plasma levels of low molecular weight proteins will filter through the glomerulus in abnormal amounts, leading to a condition known as "overflow" proteinuria. Bence-Jones proteinuria is a classic example of this type, though myoglobin and hemoglobin are also excreted in this manner (Schultze and Heremans, 1966a; Hardwicke, 1970; Hardwicke, 1974). It should be noted that increased excretion of Bence-Jones protein can cause inhibition of reabsorption of low molecular weight proteins such as α_2-microglobulin and β_2-microglobulin, resulting in a superimposed pattern of tubular proteinuria.

IV. PROTEINS IN OTHER BIOLOGICAL FLUIDS

A. Amniotic Fluid

Brock and Sutcliffe (1972) reported that elevated amniotic fluid α-fetoprotein levels could be useful in the antenatal diagnosis of fetal neural tube defects. This initial observation has been confirmed by other investigations (Allan *et al.*, 1973), and the determination of α-fetoprotein in amniotic fluid has gained widespread acceptance. Since collection of amniotic fluid involves some risk to the fetus, some authors have suggested that determination of maternal plasma α-fetoprotein be carried out as a screening procedure to identify pregnancies "at risk" (Brock *et al.*, 1973; Wald and Brock, 1974; Mildford-Ward *et al.*, 1976). Comparison studies have shown, however, that determinations of α-fetoprotein levels in maternal serum are less sensitive than amniotic fluid measurements for detection of closed defects or neural malformations in early pregnancy (Harris *et al.*, 1974; Seller *et al.*, 1974).

Currently, it is accepted that most other amniotic fluid proteins are largely maternal in origin (Johnson *et al.*, 1974; Burnett *et al.*, 1976), and recent studies have found no conclusive diagnostic significance to these determinations (Jonasson *et al.*, 1974; Haddow *et al.*, 1977). Burnett and co-workers (1976) found altered permeability to proteins in severe pre-eclampsia, but concluded that amniotic fluid protein profiles do not offer a useful clinical index of fetal status. Other groups (Jonasson *et al.*, 1974; Haddow *et al.*, 1977) have established normal ranges for amniotic fluid proteins in the hope that subsequent studies will reveal clinically significant data.

B. Synovial Fluid

The high viscosity of synovial fluid, due to its hyaluronic acid content, has presented some analytical difficulties in studying its protein content. Electrophoresis may be carried out after treatment with hyaluronidase to reduce viscosity. The electrophoretic pattern of synovial fluid can then be seen to closely resemble that of serum, the differences being a higher percentage of albumin, a lower percentage of the α_2- and γ-globulins, and a higher α_1/α_2 ratio (Schultze and Heremans, 1966d).

Investigations of specfic synovial fluid proteins have largely concentrated on inflammatory joint diseases (Pruzanski *et al.*, 1973; Bunch *et al.*, 1974; Swedlund *et al.*, 1974). The most frequently studied proteins include immunoglobulins and complement components, and attempts have been made to interpret data presented either as synovial fluid/serum protein ratios or as synovial fluid protein/synovial fluid total protein ratios.

The consistent finding of decreased complement levels in synovial fluid from patients with joint inflammation in rheumatic diseases has led to the conclusion that the complement system is an important mediator of this process (Ruddy and Colten, 1974). Bunch *et al.* (1974) have devised a method for expressing the normal range for synovial fluid complement concentration by reference to a regression line with total protein. Using this approach, they found low complement levels in patients with rheumatoid arthritis, systemic lupus erythematosus, and bacterial infections whereas other forms of synovitis gave normal results.

C. Saliva

The protein content of saliva has been determined to fall between 100 and 300 mg/dl, and these levels are affected only little by salivary stimulation (Schultze and Heremans, 1966c). Plasma proteins that have been identified in saliva include prealbumin, albumin, α_1-acid glycoprotein, α_1-antitrypsin, ceruloplasmin, β_2-macroglobulin, transferrin, β-lipo-protein, IgG, IgA, and IgM. The salivary IgA is in its dimeric secretory form with a significant amount of synthesis taking place in the salivary glands. Measurement of IgA in saliva may provide a useful laboratory guide in screening for deficiencies of the secretory immunoglobulin.

REFERENCES

Adams, D. H., and Dickinson, J. P. (1974). *Lancet* **2**, 1196–1199.

Adams, J. B., and Wacher, A. (1968). *Clin. Chim. Acta* **21**, 155–157.

Agostoni, A., Marasini, B., Stabilini, R., DelNinno, E., and Pontello, M. (1974). *Clin. Chem.* **20**, 428–429.

Agostoni, A., Del Ninno, E., Marasini, B., Colombo, M., and Stabilini, R. (1976). *In* "Protides of the Biological Fluids, Proc. 23rd. Colloquium, 1975" (H. Peeters, ed.), pp. 441–443. Pergamon, Oxford.

Alford, C. A. (1971), *Pediatr. Clin. North Am.* **18**, 99–113.

Allan, L. D., Ferguson-Smith, M. A., Donald, I., Sweet, E. M., and Gibson, A.A.M. (1973). *Lancet 2*, 522–525.

Alper, C. A. (1974). *N. Engl. J. Med.* **291**, 287–290.

Anastassea-Vlachou, C., Kattamis, C., Lagos, P., Konstantoulakis, M., and Matsaniotis, N. (1973). *Clin. Chim. Acta* **44**, 259–262.

Ansari, K. A., Wells, K., and Vatassery, G. T. (1975). *Neurology* **25**, 688–692.

Aronsen, K.-F., Ekelund, G., Kindmark, C.-D., and Laurell, C.-B. (1972). *Scand. J. Clin. Lab. Invest. Suppl.* 124, **29**, 127–136.

Barden, J., Mullinax, F., and Waller, M. (1967). *Arthritis Rheum.* **10**, 228–233.

Barratt, T. M., McLaine, P. N., and Soothill, J. F. (1970). *Arch. Dis. Child.* **45**, 496–501.

Berggard, I. (1961). *Clin. Chim. Acta* **6**, 413–429.

Berggard, I. (1970). *In* "Proteins in Normal and Pathological Urine" (Y. Manuel, J. P. Revillard, and H. Butel, eds.), pp. 7–19. Univ. Park Press, Baltimore, Maryland.

Berggard, I., and Risinger, C. (1961). *Acta Soc. Med. Ups.* **66**, 217–229.

Berggard, I., and Bearn, A. G. (1968) *J. Biol. Chem.* **243**, 4095–4103.

Berner, J. J., Ciemins, V. A., and Schroeder, E. F. (1972). *Am. J. Clin. Pathol.* **58**, 145–152.

Blainey, J. D., Brewer, D. B., Hardwicke, J., and Soothill, J. F. (1960). *Q. J. Med.* **29**, 235–256.

Bouige, D., Coudon, B., and Giraudet, P. (1973). *In* "Proceedings of the Technicon Colloquium on Automated Measurement of Proteins by Immunonephelometry," pp. 1–22. Technicon, Paris.

Boyce, W. H., King, J., and Fielden, M. (1961). *J. Clin. Invest.* **40**, 1453–1456.

Britain, C. E., Butts, J. D., and Killingsworth, L. M. (1977). *In* "Advances in Automated Analysis" (E. C. Barton *et al.*, eds.), pp. 274–277. Mediad, New York.

Brock, D. J. H., and Sutcliffe, R. G. (1972). *Lancet* **2**, 197–199.

Brock, D. J. H., Bolton, A. E., and Monaghan, J. M. (1973). *Lancet* **2**, 923–924.

Buckley, R. H., Dees, S. C., and O'Fallon, W. M. (1968). *Pediatrics* **41**, 600–611.

Bunch, T. W., Hunder, G. G., McDuffie, F. C. O'Brein, P. C., and Markowitz, H. (1974). *Mayo Clin. Proc.* **49**, 715–720.

Burnett, D., Wood, S. M., and Bradwell, A. P. (1976). *In* "Protides of the Biological Fluids, Proc. 23rd Colloquium, 1975" (H. Peeters, ed.), pp. 349–352. Pergamon, Oxford.

Butler, E. A., and Flynn, F. V. (1958). *Lancet* **2**, 978–982.

Butler, E. A., Flynn, F. V., Harris, H., and Robson, E. B. (1962). *Clin. Chim. Acta* **7**, 34–41.

Butts, W. C., James, G. E., and Keuhneman, M. (1977). *Clin. Chem.* **23**, 511–514.

Cejka, J., Mood, D. W., and Kim, C. S. (1974). *Clin. Chem.* **20**, 656–659.

Charvet, F., Manuel, Y., and Pelissier, B. (1970) *In* "Proteins in Normal and Pathological Urine" (Y. Manuel, J. P. Revillard, and H. Butel, eds.), pp. 220–223. Univ. Park Press, Baltimore, Maryland.

Claman, H. N., and Merrill, D. (1966). *J. Lab. Clin. Med.* **67**, 850–854.

Cohen, S. R., Herndon, R. M., and McKhann, G. M. (1976). *N. Engl. J. Med.* **295**, 1455–1457.

Daniels, J. C. (1975a) *In* "Serum Protein Abnormalities- Diagnostic and Clinical Aspects" (S. E. Ritzmann and J. C. Daniels, eds.), Chap. 14. Little, Brown, Boston, Massachusetts.

Daniels, J. C. (1975b) *In* "Serum Protein Abnormalities-Diagnostic and Clinical Aspects" (S. R. Ritzmann and J. C. Daniels, eds.), Chap. 15. Little, Brown, Boston, Massachusetts.

Delpech, B., and Boquet, J. (1976). *In* "Protides of the Biological Fluids, Proc. 23rd Colloquium, 1975" (H. Peeters, ed.), pp. 489–491. Pergamon, Oxford.

Dickson, I., and Alper, C. A. (1974). *Clin. Chim. Acta* **54**, 381–385.

Dillard, M. G., Pesce, A. J., Pollak, V. E., and Boreisha, I. (1971). *J. Lab. Clin. Med.* **78**, 203–215.

Ellis, D., and Buffone, G. J. (1977). *Clin. Chem.* Winston-Salem, N. C. **23**, 666–670.

Evrin, P. E., and Wibell, L. (1972). *Scand. J. Clin. Lab. Invest.* **29**, 69–74.

Felgenhauer, K., Schliep, G., and Rapic, N. (1976). *In* "Protides of the Biological Fluids, Proc. 23rd Colloquium, 1975" (H. Peeters, ed.), 481–487. Pergamon, Oxford.

Fischer, C. L., and Gill, C. W. (1975). *In* "Serum Protein Abnormalities-Diagnostic and Clinical Aspects" (S. E. Ritzmann and J. C. Daniels, eds.), pp. 331–350. Little, Brown, Boston, Massachusetts.

Fischer, C. L., Gill, C., Forrester, M., and Nakamura, R. (1976). *Am. J. Clin. Pathol.* **66**, 840–846.

Folin, O., and Denis, W. (1914). *J. Biol. Chem.* **18**, 273–277.

Forkman, B., Ganrot, P. O., Gennser, G., and Rannevik, G. (1972). *Scand. J. Clin. Lab. Invest. Suppl.* 124, **29**, 89–96.

Friberg, L. (1950). *Acta Med. Scand. Suppl.* 240, **138**, 1–124.

Ganrot, K. (1974). *Scand. J. Clin. Lab. Invest.* **34**, 75–81.

Ganrot, K., and Laurell, C.-B. (1974). *Clin. Chem.* **20**, 571–573.

Ganrot, P. O. (1972). *Scand. J. Clin. Lab. Invest. Suppl.* 124, **29**, 83–88.

Gitlin, D., and Gitlin, J. D. (1975a) *In* "The Plasma Proteins" (F. W. Putnam, ed.), Vol. II, 2nd Ed., Chap. 6. Academic Press, New York.

Gitlin, D., and Gitlin, J. D. (1975b) *In* "The Plasma Proteins" (F. W. Putnam, ed.), Vol. II, 2nd Ed., Chap. 7. Academic Press, New York.

Goel, K. M., Logan, R. W., Barnard, W. P., and Shanks, R. A. (1974). *Ann. Rheum. Dis.* **33**, 35–38.

Haddow, J. E., Macri, J. N., Munson, M., Baldwin, P., and Ritchie, R. F. (1977). *In* "Advances in Automated Analysis" (E. C. Barton *et al.*, eds.), pp. 270–273. Mediad, New York.

Hällén, J., and Laurell, C.-B. (1972). *Scand. J. Clin. Lab. Invest. Suppl.* 124, **29**, 97–103.

Hardwicke, J. (1970). *In* "The Scientific Basis of Medicine Annual Reviews." Oxford Univ. Press (Athlone), London and New York.

Hardwicke J. (1974). *In* "Protides of the Biological Fluids, Proc. 21st Colloquium, 1973" (H. Peeters, ed.), pp. 341–346. Pergamon, Oxford.

Hardwicke, J., Cameron, J. S., Harrison, J. F., Hulme, B., and Soothill, J. F. (1970). *In* "Proteins in Normal and Pathological Urine" (Y. Manuel, J. P. Revillard, and H. Butel, eds.), pp. 111–152. Univ. Park Press, Baltimore, Maryland.

Harris, R., Jennison, R. F., Barson, A. J., Lawrence, K. M., Ruoslahti, E., and Seppala, M. (1974). *Lancet* **1,** 429–433.

Heinemann, H. O., Maack, T. M., and Shennan, R. L. (1974). *Am. J. Med.* **56,** 71–82.

Hemmingsen, L., and Skaarup, P. (1975). *Scand. J. Clin. Lab Invest.* **35,** 347–353.

Henry, J. B. (1974). *In* "Clinical Diagnosis by Laboratory Methods" (I. Davidson and J. B. Henry, eds.), pp. 577–591. Saunders, Philadelphia, Pennsylvania.

Heremans, J. F., and Masson, P. L. (1973). *Clin. Chem.* **19,** 294.

Hiramatsu, S., Kojima, J., Okada, T. T., Inai, S., and Ohmori, K. (1976). *Acta Hepato-Gastroenterol.* **23,** 177–182.

Hofer, W., Misgeld, W., and Baethke, R. (1974). *In* "Protides of the Biological Fluids, Proc. 21st Colloquium, 1973" (H. Peeters, ed.), pp. 459–462. Pergamon, Oxford.

Janus, E. D., and Carrell, R. W. (1976). *In* "Protides of the Biological Fluids, Proc. 23rd Colloquium, 1975" (H. Peeters, ed.) pp. 383. Pergamon, Oxford.

Jensen, H., and Henriksen, K. (1974). *In* "Protides of the Biological Fluids, Proc. 21st Colloquium, 1973" (H. Peeters, ed.), pp. 371–374. Pergamon, Oxford.

Joachim, G. R., Cameron, S., Schwartz, M., and Becker, E. L. (1964). *J. Clin. Invest.* **43,** 2332–2346.

Johansson, B. G., Kindmark, C.-O., Trell, E. Y., and Wolheim, F. A. (1972). *Scand. J. Clin. Lab. Invest. Suppl.* 124, **29,** 117–126.

Jonasson, L. E., Evrin, P. E., and Wibell, L. (1974). *Acta Obstet. Gynecol. Scand.* **53,** 49–58.

Johnson, A. M., Umansky, I., Alper, C. A., Everett, C., and Greenspan, G. (1974). *J. Pediatc.* **84,** 588–593.

Johnson, K. P., Arrigo, S. C., Nelson, B. J., and Ginsberg, A. (1977). *Neurology* **27,** 273–277.

Kabat, E. A., Glusman, M., and Knaub, V. (1948). *Am. J. Med.* **4,** 653–662.

Kawai, T. (1973). "Clinical Aspects of the Plasma Proteins." Lippincott, Philadelphia, Pennsylvania.

Killingsworth, L. M. (1976). *In* "Protides of the Biological Fluids, Proc. 23rd Colloquium, 1975" (H. Peeters, ed.), pp. 291–294. Pergamon, Oxford.

Killingsworth, L. M. (1978). *Clin. Chem.* **24,** 728.

Killingsworth, L. M., Britain, C. E., and Woodard, L. L. (1975a). *Clin. Chem.* Winston-Salem, N.C. **21,** 1465–1468.

Killingsworth, L. M., Young, W. J., and Roberts, J. E. (1975b). *Clin. Chem.* Winston-Salem, N.C. **21,** 1921.

Kindmark, C.-O. (1976) *In* "Protides of the Biological Fluids, Proc. 23rd Colloquium, 1975" (H. Peeters, ed.), pp. 431–435. Pergamon, Oxford.

Kindmark, C.-O., and Laurell, C.-B. (1972). *Scand. J. Clin. Lab. Invest. Suppl.* 124, **29,** 105–115.

Lambert, P. P., Gassee, J. P., and Askenasi, R. (1970). *In* "Proteins in Normal and Pathological Urine" (Y. Manuel, J. P. Revillard, and H. Butel, eds.), pp. 67–82. Univ. Park Press, Baltimore, Maryland.

Lamoureux, G., Jolicoeur, R., Giard, N., St-Hilaire, M., and Duplantis, F. (1975). *Neurology* **25,** 537–546.

Laterre, E. C., and Manuel, Y. (1970). *In* "Proteins in Normal and Pathological Urine" (Y. Manuel, J. P. Revillard, and H. Butel, eds.), pp. 172–187. Univ. Park Press, Baltimore, Maryland.

Laterre, E. C., Callewaert, A., Heremans, J. F., and Sfaello, Z. (1970). *Neurology* **20**, 982–990.

Laurell, C.-B. (1972a). *Scand. J. Clin. Lab. Invest. Suppl.* 124, **29**, 71–82.

Laurell, C.-B. (1972b). *Scand. J. Clin. Lab Invest.* **30**, 233–235.

Laurell, C.-B. (1973). *Clin. Chem.* **19**, 99–102.

Link, H. (1973). *Clin. Chim. Acta* **46**, 383–389.

Link, H., and Muller, R. (1971). *Arch. Neurol.* **25**, 326–344.

LoGrippo, G. A., Anselm, K., and Hayashi, H. (1971). *Am. J. Gastroenterol.* **56**, 357–363.

Lyngbye, J., and Krøll, J. (1971). *Clin. Chem.* Winston-Salem, N.C. **17**, 495–500.

MacLean, P. R., and Robson (1967). *Lancet* **1**, 539–542.

MacSween, R. N. M., Horne, C. H. W., Moffat, A. J., and Hughes, H. M. (1972). *J. Clin. Pathol.* **25**, 789–792.

Maiorca, R. Scarpioni, L., Cambi, W., Carrara, G. C., and Dall'aglio, P. (1967). *Clin. Chim. Acta* **16**, 253–257.

Milford-Ward, A. (1976). *In* "Protides of the Biological Fluids, Proc. 23rd Colloquium, 1975" (H. Peeters, ed.), pp. 353–357. Pergamon, Oxford.

Müller-Eberhard, H. J. (1975). *In* "The Plasma Proteins" (F. W. Putnam, ed.), Vol. I, Chap. 8. Academic Press, New York.

Norman, M. E., Gall, E. P., Taylor, A., Laster, L., and Nilsson, U. R. (1975). *J. Pediatr.* **87**, 912–916.

O'Toole, R. D., Thornton, G. F., Mukherjee, M. K., and Neogy, N. N. (1971). *Arch. Neurol.* **25**, 218–224.

Owen, J. A. (1967). *Adv. Clin. Chem.* **9**, 1–41.

Perry, J. J., Bray, P. F., and Hackett, T. N. (1974). *Clin. Chem.* Winston-Salem, N.C. **20**, 1441–1443.

Peters, T. (1975). *In* "The Plasma Proteins" (F. W. Putnam, ed.), Vol. I, 2nd Ed., Chap. 3. Academic Press, New York.

Peterson, P. A., Evrin, P. E., and Berggard, I. (1969). *J. Clin. Invest.* **48**, 1189–1198.

Poortmans, J. R. (1970). *In* "Proteins in Normal and Pathological Urine" (Y. Manuel, J. P. Revillard, and H. Butel, eds.), pp. 229–234. Univ. Park Press, Baltimore, Maryland.

Poortmans, J. R. (1974). *In* "Protides of the Biological Fluids, Proc. 21st Colloquium, 1973" (H. Peeters, ed.), pp. 375–378. Pergamon, Oxford.

Poortmans, J., and Jeanloz, R. W. (1968). *J. Clin. Invest.* **47**, 386–393.

Poulik, M. D., and Weiss, M. L. (1975). *In* "The Plasma Proteins" (F. W. Putnam, ed.), Vol. I, 2nd Ed., Chap. 2. Academic Press, New York.

Pruzanski, W., Russell, M. L., Gordon, D. A., and Ogryzlo, M. A. (1973). *Am. J. Med.* **265**, 483–490.

Putnam, F. W. (1975a). *In* "The Plasma Proteins" (F. W. Putnam, ed.), Vol. I, 2nd Ed., Chap 1. Academic Press, New York.

Putnam, F. W. (1975b). *In* "The Plasma Proteins" (F. W. Putnam, ed.), Vol. I, 2nd Ed., Chap. 6. Academic Press, New York.

Quittner, H. (1974). *Ann. Clin. Lab. Sci.* **4**, 471.

Ravnskov, U., and Johansson, B. G. (1974). *In* "Protides of the Biological Fluids, Proc. 21st Colloquium, 1973" (H. Peeters, ed.), pp. 513–517. Pergamon, Oxford.

Revillard, J. P., Fries, D., Salle, B., Blanc, N., and Traeger, J. (1970a). *In* "Proteins in Normal and Pathological Urine" (Y. Manuel, J. P. Revillard, and H. Butel, eds.), pp. 188–197. Univ. Park Press, Baltimore, Maryland.

Revillard, J. P., Manuel, Y., Francois, R., and Traeger, J. (1970b). *In* "Proteins in Normal and Pathological Urine" (Y. Manuel, J. P. Revillard, and H. Butel, eds.), pp. 209–219. Univ. Park Press, Baltimore, Maryland.

Ricanti, E. S., and Hall, P. W. (1974). *In* "Protides of the Biological Fluids, Proc. 21st Colloquium, 1973" (H. Peeters, ed.), pp. 357–361. Pergamon, Oxford.

Riddoch, D., and Thompson, R. A. (1970). *Brit. Med. J.* **1**, 396–399.

Ritchie, R. F. (1974a) *In* "Protides of the Biological Fluids, Proc. 21st Colloquium, 1973" (H. Peeters, ed.), pp. 593–603. Pergamon, Oxford.

Ritchie, R. F. (1974b). *Patient Care (May)*, 2–7.

Ritzmann, S. E. (1975). *In* "Serum Protein Abnormalities-Diagnostic and Clinical Aspects" (S. E. Ritzmann and J. C. Daniels, eds.) Chap. 19. Little, Brown, Boston, Massachusetts.

Robinson, R. R. (1970). *In* "Proteins in Normal and Pathological Urine" (Y. Manuel, J. P. Revillard, and H. Butel, eds.), pp. 224–228. Univ. Park Press, Baltimore, Maryland.

Rowe, D. S., and Soothill, J. F. (1961). *Clin. Sci.* **21**, 75–85.

Ruddy, S., and Colten, H. R. (1974). *N. Engl. J. Med.* **290**, 1284–1288.

Savory, J., and Heintges, M. G. (1973). *Neurology* **23**, 953–958.

Scherer, R., and Ruhenstroth-Bauer, G. (1976). *Clin. Chim. Acta* **66**, 417–433.

Schliep, G., and Felgenhauer, K. (1974). *J. Neurol.* **207**, 171–181.

Schneck, S. A., and Claman, H. N. (1969). *Arch. Neurol.* **20**, 132–139.

Schultze, H. E., and Heremans, J. F. (1966a). "Molecular Biology of Human Proteins, Nature and Metabolism of Extracellular Proteins" Vol. I, Sec. IV, Chap. 2. Elsevier, Amsterdam.

Schultze, H. E., and Heremans, J. F. (1966b). "Molecular Biology of Human Proteins Nature and Metabolism of Extracellular Proteins," Vol. 1, Sec. IV, Chap. 3, Elsevier, Amsterdam.

Schultze, H. E., and Heremans, J. F. (1966c). "Molecular Biology of Human Proteins, Nature and Metabolism of Extracellular Proteins" Vol. 1, Sec. IV, Chap. 4. Elsevier, Amsterdam.

Schultze, H. E., and Heremans, J. F. (1966d). "Molecular Biology of Human Proteins, Nature and Metabolism of Extracellular Proteins" Vol. 1, Sec. IV, Chap. 9. Elsevier, Amsterdam.

Seller, M. J., Singer, J. D., Coltart, T. M., and Campbell, S. (1974). *Lancet* **1**, 428–429.

Skrabanek, P., Staunton, H., Holland, P. D. J., and Lawlor, L. (1973). *J. Ir. Med. Assoc.* **66**, 692–696.

Smith, H., Bannister, B., and O'Shea, M. J. (1973). *Lancet* **2**, 591–593.

Smith, S. J., Bos, G., Esseveld, M. R., Van Eijk, H. G., and Gerbrandy, J. (1977). *Clin. Chim. Acta* **81**, 75–85.

Statland, B. E., Winkel, P., and Killingsworth, L. M., (1976). *Clin. Chem.* **22**, 1635–1638.

Stuhlinger, W., Gabl, F., Asamer, H., and Dittrich, P. (1974). *In* "Protides of the Biological Fluids, Proc. 21st Colloquium, 1973" (H. Peeters, ed.), pp. 453–456). Pergamon, Oxford.

Sun, T., Lien, Y. Y., and Gross, S. (1978). *Ann. Clin Lab. Sci.* **8**, 219–227.

Swedlund, H. A., Hunder, G. G., and Gleich, J. (1974). *Ann. Rheum. Dis.* **33**, 162–164.

Tourtellotte, W. W., Tavalato, B., Parker, J. A., and Comiso, P. (1971). *Arch. Neurol.* **25**, 345–350.

Trip, J. A. J., Arisz, L., Van der Hem, G. K., and Mandema, E. (1968). *Clin. Chim. Acta* **20**, 479–486.

Tucker, E. S. and Nakamura, R. M. (1975). *In* "Serum Protein Abnormalities-Diagnostic and Clinical Aspects" (S. E. Ritzmann and J. C. Daniels, eds.), Chap. 16. Little, Brown, Boston, Massachusetts.

Veys, E. M., and Claessens, H. E. (1968). *Ann. Rheum. Dis.* **27**, 431–439.

Wald, N. H., and Brock, D. J. H. (1974). *Lancet* **1**, 765–767.

Watkins, J., Milford-Ward, A., White, P. A. E., and Swannell, A. J. (1976). *In* "Protides of the Biological Fluids, Proc. 23rd Colloquium, 1975" (H. Peeters, ed.), pp. 455–459. Pergamon, Oxford.

Weeke, E. O. B. (1974). *In* "Protides of the Biological Fluids, Proc. 21st Colloquium, 1973" (H. Peeters, ed.), pp. 363–369. Pergamon, Oxford.

Weeke, B., and Jarnum, S. (1971). *Gut* **12**, 297–302.

Weeke, B., and Krasilnikoff, P. A. (1971). *In* "Protides of the Biological Fluids, Proc. 18th Colloquium, 1970" (H. Peeters, ed.), pp. 173–179. Pergamon, Oxford.

Weeke, B., and Krasilnikoff, P. A. (1972). *Acta Med. Scand.* **192**, 149–155.

Weeke, B., Weeke, E., and Bendixen, G. (1971a). *Acta Med. Scand.* **189**, 113–118.

Weeke, B., Weeke, E., and Bendixen, G. (1971b). *Acta Med. Scand.* **189**, 119–123.

Weiss, D. L. (1975). *Ann. Clin. Lab. Sci.* **5**, 363–368.

Werner, M. (1969). *Clin. Chim. Acta* **25**, 299–305.

Whicher, J. T. (1978). *Clin. Chem.* **24**, 7–22.

Wibell, L., and Evrin, P. E. (1974). *In* "Protides of the Biological Fluids, Proc. 21st Colloquium, 1973" (H. Peeters, ed.), pp. 519–523. Pergamon, Oxford.

Winkel, P., Statland, B. E., and Nielsen, M. K. (1976). *Scand. J. Clin. Lab. Invest.* **36**, 531–537.

Index